PRAISE FOR Ma

"This book is a love letter to the womb, general. It is a lifeline back to a positive relationship with our bodies. *Magic Within* is a book written for all women to connect with womb energy, regardless of their physical circumstances. It is a reminder that no external force is stronger than the power of a woman's body. You will find whole body healing through the words in this book."

—Phoenix Lefae, author of *Witches, Heretics & Warrior Women*

"I love Rhoda's voice in this intimate and supportive book. It feels like having a nurturing womb-side chat with a best friend, sister, or auntie who can guide you through the Womb Rites that were once natural to our ancient cultures. It's vital that we all learn how powerful the womb is as the source of life, death, and rebirth. Once you awaken your womb, you will reconnect to your innate magic within."

—Seren Bertrand, co-author of *Womb Awakening* and
    Magdalene Mysteries, author of *Spirit Weaver*

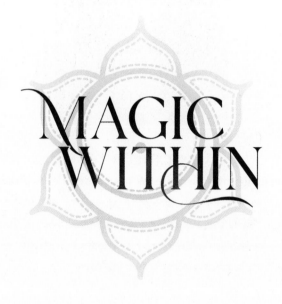

MAGIC WITHIN

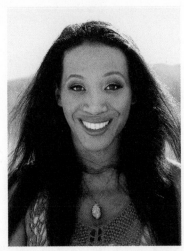

ABOUT THE AUTHOR

Rhoda Jordan Shapiro has worked for over a decade as a tantric educator, training women to step into their power by way of meditation, movement, dance, and yoga. She is the author of *Fierce Woman*, and the founder and editor in chief of *The Milpitas Beat*, a local newspaper. She lives in the San Francisco Bay Area with her husband and two children.

RHODA JORDAN SHAPIRO

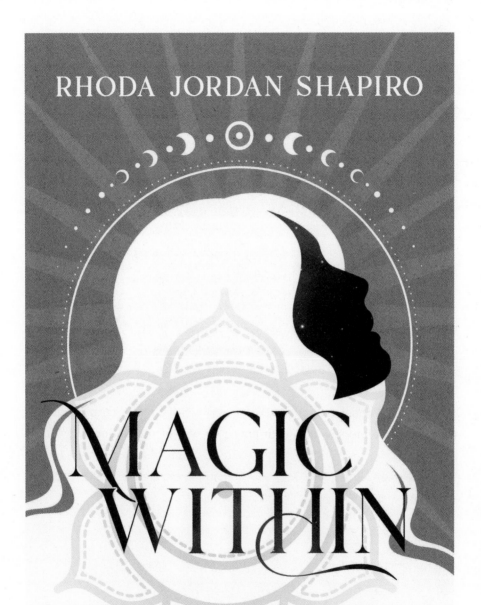

MAGIC WITHIN

*Womb-Centered Wisdom to Realize
the Power of Your Sacred Feminine Self*

Llewellyn Publications
Woodbury, Minnesota

FIRST EDITION
First Printing, 2023

Book design by R. Brasington
Cover design by Cassie Willett

Llewellyn Publications is a registered trademark of Llewellyn Worldwide Ltd.

Library of Congress Cataloging-in-Publication Data (Pending)
ISBN: 978-0-7387-7179-3

Llewellyn Worldwide Ltd. does not participate in, endorse, or have any authority or responsibility concerning private business transactions between our authors and the public.

All mail addressed to the author is forwarded but the publisher cannot, unless specifically instructed by the author, give out an address or phone number.

Any internet references contained in this work are current at publication time, but the publisher cannot guarantee that a specific location will continue to be maintained. Please refer to the publisher's website for links to authors' websites and other sources.

Llewellyn Publications
A Division of Llewellyn Worldwide Ltd.
2143 Wooddale Drive
Woodbury, MN 55125-2989
www.llewellyn.com

Printed in the United States of America

OTHER BOOKS BY RHODA JORDAN SHAPIRO

Fierce Woman

This one is for my ancestors.
My story would be nonexistent,
if not for their stories.

CONTENTS

EXERCISES

INTRODUCTION

The first time I started to pay my womb any kind of attention at all was when I was pregnant with my first child. Suddenly I had this overwhelming urge to place my hands over my womb all the time, to feel and connect with the life growing inside of me. I couldn't even begin to comprehend the magic of it.

Some nights, I'd lie awake in bed beside my husband, just feeling and breathing into my womb, that deep sense of connection lulling me off to sleep. I had never experienced anything quite like it before.

From that point on, I was hooked. The relationship with my womb had been forged. Even after giving birth to my baby, I continued to find myself drawn to my womb, hypnotized by the comforting yet strong feeling I would get inside of me whenever I held it or focused on it.

Why is this? I wondered.

While I was pregnant, I had assumed that it had been the excitement of creating life that had entranced me. But once the baby was out, I realized it was more than that.

My womb carried *power*. And it wasn't something that simply started and ended with pregnancy and childbirth. Although I was just starting to notice it, that power in my womb had always been there inside of me. This realization would set me off on a journey of deeply awakening my womb and reclaiming my power, self-love, and sensuality in the process.

For many women, there is no strong feeling of connection with the womb. Each and every day, our precious energy is siphoned off to attend to a million different details, and oftentimes, our wombs just aren't on our radar. We pay very little, if any, attention to our wombs. This sets the stage for some major disconnect, separating us from truly knowing ourselves and the pure potential we hold.

Why is this so important, anyway? Why is awareness of your womb such a game changer?

Well, for starters, a womb has the ability to nurture and create life. It doesn't get any more powerful than that. Your womb is full of creative potential that can be used toward empowering every aspect of your life—career, money, relationships, sex, spiritual fulfillment, self-love, manifestation, wellness. The force of the womb is all-encompassing, and it's something you can dip into anytime you need it.

Owning your womb power means owning every facet of your life. You start to feel at home and at ease in your own body. The busy chatter of the mind starts to drop away, allowing a radiant inner clarity to take its place. You begin moving, speaking, and thinking as your truest, most potent self. The real you. The one who's not here to simply go through the motions, but rather the one who knows the way to deep fulfillment is to live the life that is calling you from within—the life that others will tell you is impossible.

But nothing is impossible when you open up to the magic your body holds.

This book was written to remind you of who you are and what you contain within. Your womb holds the key to your greatest joy and potential. It is your inner compass. It carries your wisdom and your wildness. It houses the whispers of your deepest desires and emotions. Through it, your inner and outer worlds are illuminated. The womb is every woman's direct route to unlimited creativity, sensuality, energy, pleasure, and purpose.

But let's ground ourselves for a moment here. I don't want to sugarcoat this. It might sound awesome to own your womb power, but at the same time, untangling the mysteries of your womb won't be all sunshine and roses. Our wombs have been hit hard. Throughout history, women's hopes, dreams, and bodies have been crushed, all in pursuit of upholding a world that has, in many ways, looked at the feminine as inferior.

Every woman has undergone her share of heartaches and struggles. We all know what it feels like to experience grief, loss, and pain. When we have unresolved feelings and emotions, they don't merely dissipate. They linger in the body, burrowing themselves into our cells and organs. The womb in particular can carry many emotional memories, holding space for all that is unprocessed until the moment we're ready to deal with things.

So, the promise of this womb journey might sound intriguing, but at the same time, know that it could potentially challenge you in the process. As you explore and understand your womb more deeply, you will also be healing. You might need to go slow and take baby steps. And that's all perfectly fine. Do what feels right to you. You can never go wrong if you listen to what your body truly needs.

The pages in this book were written to seduce you into remembering who you are: a wildly powerful, creative, sexy, fierce, loving, and vibrant goddess who is meant to love and live this life to the absolute fullest.

Even if you don't have a physical womb in your body, you can still partake in the practices and benefit from this book. If you've had a hysterectomy and no longer have a womb, this book is also for you. You are not lacking at all when it comes to being a woman and stepping into your womb power. The power of the womb is an energy, and regardless of whether the womb is physically there or not, it can still be aligned to.

Something that is also important to mention: this book has been written for all who identify as women; this means that trans women are also encouraged to read these pages and become more intimately aware of their feminine energies. I truly believe that it's vital to offer these practices to *all* women who want to go deeper into exploring and understanding who they are and what kind of power they hold.

There are exercises in this book that specifically revolve around focusing on the womb or breasts. If you don't physically have a womb or breasts, you can substitute your focus to your lower abdomen or your chest. If a specific practice calls for you to focus on your vagina and you don't have one, you can use the pelvic region.

At present, this world does not fully comprehend the sacredness of our feminine bodies and natures. Our wombs are undergoing a kind of crisis right now. Many women are struggling with things like anxiety, depression, stress, lack of self-love, low confidence, shame, guilt, body dysmorphia, and loneliness. It can often feel like everything is beyond our control, that there's nothing we can do to improve and empower our own lives.

But there is something.

That something is calling you, daring you, to surrender to the awesomeness that you naturally have within. The more attention you pay your womb, the more attention your womb will pay back to you. And once that relationship begins, life will never be the same.

As you dive into these pages, I highly recommend you use a specific notebook or journal that is solely dedicated to the journey of exploring your own womb magic within. In your Womb Journal, you can write about your experiences as you go through the many rituals and practices in this book.

Before you go on to chapter 1, take some time to do a quick ritual. Place both hands on the womb, just below the navel. Send love to your womb in the form of a deep inhale. Feel that love entering and connecting with the womb. And when you exhale, let the womb relax.

That power. Do you feel it?

You have it in you. The power to heal, to transform, to love, to shine, to live the kind of joyful life that grabs hold of the soul and never lets go.

The secret to all that has been under your nose, *literally,* this whole time.

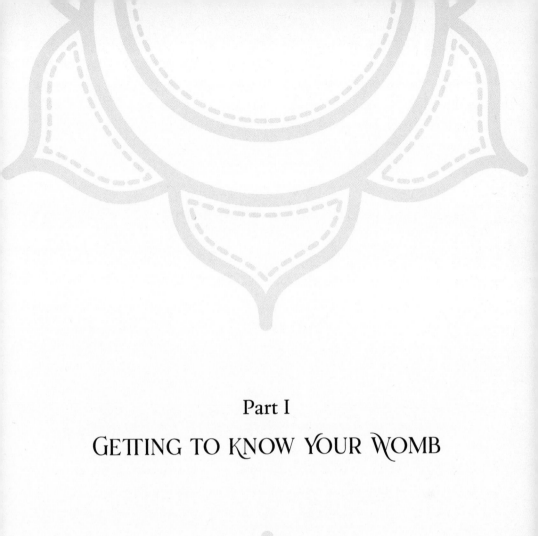

Part I

GETTING TO KNOW YOUR WOMB

Chapter 1

THE POWER OF YOUR WOMB

"Womb energy is simultaneously the most powerful
and most neglected force in the universe."
    —Abiola Abrams[1]

When I was a young girl, I knew nothing about my womb and the power it held. No one ever pulled me aside and broke it down for me. I, like many girls growing up, was oblivious to the potential I carried within. I knew we could make babies, and that getting my period was a step in that direction. But that was about it. That was the full extent of my knowledge when it came to the womb.

It wasn't until I was an adult, pregnant with my first child, that I started to understand just how powerful my womb really was. But it doesn't have to take pregnancy or childbirth to become acquainted with our wombs and the power they hold. That was just the beginning of my womb adventure, the turning point that set me off on an ever-unfolding journey of inner exploration.

Maybe your womb adventure is beginning right now, just by reading this book. Or maybe you're already in the middle of your womb adventure and looking for the next part of it. Regardless of who you are and what your story is, this book was written *just for you*. Every woman deserves to know about the power inherent in her womb and body.

---

1. Abiola Abrams, *African Goddess Initiation* (New York: Hay House, 2021), 356.

When a woman heals and awakens her womb, she can:

- Heal unhealthy past relationships
- Fall in love with her body and herself
- Feel more energy and vibrancy
- Release shame
- Experience awe-inspiring orgasms
- Experience more pleasure and intimacy during sex
- Heal issues related to pregnancy and childbirth
- Unleash her creative abilities
- Gain confidence and activate her inner power
- Restore wellness to her reproductive organs
- Stop menstrual pain or discomfort
- Release stuck emotions
- Rid herself of energies from toxic past lovers
- End disempowering patterns or habits
- Strengthen her mental health
- Feel at ease in her own body
- Surrender to the "flow" of her own life

YOUR WOMB IS A POWER SOURCE

For centuries now, the power in our wombs has been used against us. Take ancient Greece, for instance. In those times, people came up with some pretty astounding achievements in philosophy, astronomy, and architecture. But when it came to understanding women, some doctors from ancient Greek times were completely clueless. During that period, doctors believed in what became known as "the wandering womb," where the womb would just randomly disappear from where it was supposed to be and move throughout the body. They used this wandering womb theory to explain why women were so different from men. Basically, they blamed the womb whenever they thought a woman was showing signs of mental imbalance or having a physical issue.

The Greek word for the womb is *hystera*, which is where the word *hysteria* actually originated from. So back then, when a woman would "act up," hysteria via wandering womb would be the diagnosis.

This wandering womb theory persisted for hundreds of years in European medicine, but eventually was discarded in favor of, you know, reality and science and all that. Luckily, that particular belief is behind us now, and the womb is no longer accused of wandering. But there are still many other battles to fight.

No matter what's happening or how far we've come, society is still finding all the ways in which to justify classifying women as crazy, emotional, unbalanced, dramatic, weak, not good enough, not strong enough, not beautiful enough…it's a long list, and I know you get the picture.

As I'm sitting here writing this, the US Supreme Court has just overturned *Roe v. Wade*, putting an end to the constitutional right to abortion, which had been in place for nearly half a century. Our world seems fixated on dictating what women do with their bodies and wombs. And when it comes to the medical field, don't even get me started. Countless women have endured unnecessary surgeries involving the womb.

Today, the cesarean section is the most common surgery among women in the United States. In the last year alone, the World Health Organization has found that one in five births is a cesarean section, and they expect that a third of births will soon happen via C-section.[2]

Not surprisingly, the second most common surgery among women is the hysterectomy. Removing our wombs has become something of a trend, happening to a total of ten out of one hundred thousand women. And it's happening to Black women at an even higher rate.

Why exactly is this happening?

It could be because our doctors aren't versed in the ways of understanding, healing, and nurturing the womb, and so they rush toward prescribing one

---

2. World Health Organization, "Caesarean section rates continue to rise, amid growing inequalities in access," World Health Organization, June 16, 2021, https://www.who.int/news/item/16-06-2021-caesarean-section-rates-continue-to-rise-amid-growing-inequalities-in-access.

of the only options they know: surgery. Western medicine has only thought about the womb in regard to pregnancy and childbirth—anything beyond that simply doesn't exist. If a woman comes in with a womb that is in desperate need of healing, chances are her doctor won't be whipping out the herbs and hot water for a soothing yoni steam. Nor will that doctor come anywhere close to uttering words like *womb wrapping* or making recommendations for foods and supplements that facilitate womb health. It simply doesn't happen. And if it does, it's extremely rare.

This isn't meant to be a harsh criticism on doctors or Western medicine. A surgeon literally saved my life in 2018 after a terrible emergency that actually stemmed from my C-section. (More on that later.)

And, of course, there are many women whose lives depended on having that hysterectomy, and whose babies' lives were saved by cesarean. In some cases, there really weren't any other options aside from surgery.

If you have experienced a hysterectomy and no longer have a physical womb, just know that this does nothing to take away from the power you carry within. Although your womb isn't there physically, the space in your body still holds on to that power. You will always have it with you, no matter what. However, when you do undergo a C-section, hysterectomy, or any other surgery involving your reproductive organs, the body needs to be nurtured back into balance.

When the womb is physically cut into, it experiences a great deal of trauma and pain. In order to heal, women must take actions to restore the womb back to its natural vitality. And if the womb has been removed, women can still work to heal the area in which it used to reside. The problem is that many women aren't aware that this process is necessary, and usually only focus on the appearance of the scar on the surface, not realizing that on the inside, healing of a deeper magnitude is much needed.

And it isn't just the trauma of surgery that can bring imbalance into one's womb. It's also things like:

- Stuck emotions
- Sexual abuse

- Toxic relationships
- Miscarriage
- Stillbirth
- Abortion
- Body shame
- Birth trauma
- Lack of self-love

Any major event that happens in a woman's body must be acknowledged, understood, and, if needed, healed. Our wombs carry the imprints of past lovers, relationships, and sexual hurts. Some of us carry these imprints around for years, wondering why we feel so off-balance or numb to our bodies. When we're not conscious of what's happening within our feminine landscape, this is when physical imbalances in our wombs may start to take shape. It's no wonder our rates of hysterectomy and other womb issues are so high.

As a result of holding on to these past imprints in the womb, some women may also find they feel disconnected from their natural vitality, turned off by the idea of having sex, or even caught in cycles where they're stuck in unhealthy relationships.

Not only does the womb nurture and create, but it's also a place that absorbs feelings and emotions in a woman's body. Any form of emotional imbalance, grief, sadness, or negativity will be held by the womb, until we're ready to release it.

When we begin the work of healing and connecting with our wombs, we can help our bodies release any negative emotions and past experiences. We can come back to ourselves, to who we're truly meant to be in this world. We're all powerful women. If we can surrender to the magic that is in our womb space, we can use that magic to color and enliven every area of our lives.

To first begin the journey toward womb wellness, we have to understand exactly what makes our wombs so powerful. Why are they so sacred and essential? And why isn't this something that's discussed as much as it should be in our world?

THE WOMB'S POWER

A few thousand years ago, an ancient Indian text known as the Rigveda was written. In it, *hiranyagarbha*, which is a Sanskrit word that translates to "golden womb," is mentioned. This golden womb is known as the source of creation from which the entire universe manifested. And it isn't just ancient India where the womb's power was understood. Knowledge of the womb's significance can be found in indigenous cultures and ancient texts all over the world. The Egyptian's power symbol, known as the ankh, is said by many to be a representation of the womb itself.

If you think about it, the world is really one great, big, cosmic womb. The energy of that cosmic womb is present everywhere, and within all of us, including men.

In Japanese culture, there is a word, *hara*, which is believed to be where our energy force originates from. No matter the gender of the individual, the hara can be found in the belly or womb area. In Chinese Medicine and Taoism, this point is known as the lower *dantian*, and it's also believed that a person's personal power originates from this area. The lower dantian is the focal point for many forms of marital arts, meditation, and other practices. As the hara and dantian correspond to the womb area, this means that every gender has the ability to tap into womb power.

Not to mention, we all have our beginnings in the womb, and even as we emerge from it and go out into the world, that womb energy is always with us. The cosmic womb, or golden womb, is always in direct connection to our own wombs.

If this is hard to imagine, try to picture a mother. After she gives birth to her children and they move out of her body and into the physical world, the connection between them still remains. The bond is always there, and will never be broken, no matter what. It's like that with the cosmic womb as well. The cosmic womb is the Mother, and the wombs we carry are the children to that Mother. Regardless of what happens, this connection, this ability to tap into source, into the universal, will be forever present. I don't know about you, but to me, it's comforting to know I've got this direct line to the cosmic at all times.

If we look back, we can find many traces of ancient cultures and their reverence for the womb. Back then, the womb's power was just a given. Today, not so much. In our patriarchal society, we've disconnected from this innate wisdom, and instead have looked outside of ourselves for fulfillment, pleasure, and happiness.

What others think of us, the amount of social media followers we have, the kinds of material items we own—we've allowed these kinds of superficial things to dictate our focus. And in doing so, we've distanced ourselves from trusting our intuition, our inner wisdom, and our voice. Looking outside of ourselves for happiness is never anything but a recipe for disaster. And yet we repeat this practice over and over again.

By establishing a connection with your womb, you are connecting to the blazing truth that lies within you. You are actively embracing the beauty, pleasure, creativity, and self-love that is your birthright. And when this happens, you start to free-fall into a deep state of joy that will not be fleeting like all the other times, that will not be dependent on any romantic partnership, or any social media platform, or any amount of online retail therapy.

Not knowing your own power is the ultimate betrayal against yourself. You must make it your mission to know yourself as sacred, lovable, and capable of accomplishing whatever is in your heart.

You don't have to continue conforming or struggling to be someone you're not just to make others around you feel comfortable. First of all, that's way too much work and effort. And second of all, owning your womb power is as simple as taking your next breath.

How Did We Get Here?!

Something I used to wonder about all the time is how, exactly, we got here. And by here, I mean, this place where we've forgotten our power. Where we've forgotten who we are. It's like humankind has experienced this sort of collective amnesia that's doing nothing but holding us back.

When I discovered just how much power and sacredness I held in my womb and body, I have to admit, I was kind of upset! Okay, well, first I got really excited and jumped up and down like a kid. But after I sobered up and got to thinking, I started to get seriously upset about the ways in which humanity has forgotten itself. It has neglected to uphold women as powerful, worthy, and capable leaders whose contributions are valued in the world.

Our technological advancements and economic vitality are looked at as signs of evolution and triumph. There's no doubt that a neanderthal from one hundred thousand years ago would look at this new world in awe and wonder. But although these kinds of advancements over the years have been quite impressive, we need to stop and ask ourselves this: How much ground have we made when it comes to advancing our understanding of ourselves as sacred, precious, and powerful beings who are capable of things we can't even begin to imagine yet?

Some scholars believe that thousands of years ago, many past civilizations were built around feminine leadership. However, as time went on, the balance shifted, and the patriarchy began to set in. Today, we are still caught in this disappointing cycle where women are seen and treated as "less than." It's no wonder many women hold back their magic, afraid to take up too much space and stand in their power.

We can look back in time at all the womb carvings and depictions and get smatterings of ancient wisdom, realizing all the potential we hold. We can also actually feel this potential within. As we dive deeper into this book, I'll be sharing lots of practices and techniques for nurturing your womb and bringing its power up to the surface, where it can be felt and expressed. Some of what I'm sharing is tantric in nature. It comes from my years of learning, teaching, and exploring sacred practices that originated in India several thousand years ago. Tantra is a yogic path that uses the breath, sound, movement, and visualization to bring you into harmony with the body and open your natural vitality. This is the foundation for the work in this book.

I've also devoted time to studying the ancient practices of my ancestors and how they nurtured and cared for the womb. I looked to Africa and Asia, where my ancestors originated from, and learned the ways of vaginal steaming and womb wellness. I gathered all the most potent and powerful practices that I use personally, and that I've shared with various students of mine over the years. I truly feel that knowing these practices can support you in being the truest and best version of yourself.

It does you no good to keep your power hidden. You are meant to shine, to be a bearer of light amid the darkness. The power you hold inside of your womb is precious. You can direct this power into relationships, projects, missions, and revolutions that will drastically alter this planet in positive and impactful ways.

WOMBATOMY

Before we get into the practices, let's lay some groundwork by understanding a little more about the womb …

Womb

The womb has the ability to stretch and expand beyond its normal size. On average, the womb is a mere three inches in length and two inches in width. Make a fist, and that'll give you some idea of the womb's size. It's located in the pelvic area, between the bladder and rectum. During pregnancy, the womb can expand to the size of a watermelon to accommodate the growing baby within it.

Another word for womb is *uterus*. The womb, or uterus, is connected to the fallopian tubes and ovaries. At the bottom of the womb is the cervix, which connects the vagina to the womb. All these feminine parts carry tremendous power and are in need of your love and attention. When you start to take care of these parts of yourself, you'll notice the difference in how you feel, move, think, and speak. Reclaiming these parts of yourself is a potent practice, a way of stepping into your power.

Fallopian Tubes

The fallopian tubes are two long, thin tubes that extend from the ovaries to the uterus. They're also known as uterine tubes or oviducts, and they are each about four to five inches long. Eggs move from ovaries to uterus through these slender tubes, which contain several different layers within. Present inside these layers is cilia. With its hairlike structure, cilia move the ovulated egg through the fallopian tubes to the uterus. Fertilization usually occurs in the fallopian tubes.

Ovaries

The ovaries are located on either side of the uterus. We've got two of them, just as we do fallopian tubes. The ovaries carry eggs that are released for reproduction. They also secrete hormones like estrogen and progesterone, which work to launch puberty and menopause into motion and to also nurture a regular menstrual cycle. Although the ovaries look bigger in illustrations, each one is actually only about the size and shape of an almond.

One of the most fascinating things about the ovaries is that when a baby girl is born, she already carries hundreds of thousands to millions of eggs inside her ovaries. This means that a baby girl is born with all the eggs she'll ever have in her entire life. This is different from boys, who aren't born with sperm cells; those get produced later, starting with puberty. So, if you think about it, when a mother is carrying a baby girl within her womb, she is carrying the makings of her potential grandchildren within her as well.

Cervix

The cervix is positioned at the bottom of the womb. It's shaped like a tube, and it connects uterus to vagina. It's only about two inches long, but it widens during labor so that the baby can get out. When we menstruate, it's the cervix that's allowing for the release of menstrual blood. The cervix also produces mucus, which helps sperm travel through the fallopian tubes.

Vagina

The vagina is known as an elastic, muscular canal or tube that is between the cervix and vulva. It's basically what connects our wombs to the world outside our bodies. At the opening of the vagina is the vulva, and on the interior end is the cervix. Many times, people confuse the vagina with the vulva, which is on the outside. The vagina is actually the part on the inside. Just like the cervix, the vagina can stretch and expand, which is extremely vital for moving the baby out during childbirth. It's also the place used for insertion, like with a penis, tampons, or menstrual cups.

Vulva

The vulva is what you see on the outside. It's the external parts of a woman's genitalia, which includes the clitoris, labia, and vaginal opening.

THERE'S A DEEPER WAY

Although these feminine parts of our bodies are known as making up the reproductive system, don't let those words inhibit you from understanding that there is a deeper way to connect to these aspects of our feminine selves. The magic of our wombs, ovaries, fallopian tubes, cervixes, vulvas, and vaginas is much more than a system based in offspring reproduction.

If we can start thinking of them, connecting to them, and understanding them as more than what society tells us, we can start to embrace ourselves and our bodies in new, exciting ways. The organs in our feminine reproductive systems are sacred and require our love, energy, and focus.

WOMB JOURNAL

The beauty of journaling lies in its simplicity. When you're trying to process and understand things that are happening in your life, journaling is a great tool for that. It's also perfect for documenting your life journey and capturing certain moments and experiences that might otherwise be forgotten.

I highly encourage you to start your own Womb Journal. This journal would essentially be your place to write about your experiences with your womb and all the practices we'll be diving into throughout the book. A Womb

Journal is also a place to write about emotions, creativity, romantic relationships, sex, pregnancy, childbirth, body image, and menstruation; all those areas relate to the womb and can offer great ways of understanding where you're at and what you need during your journey.

If you do decide to grab a journal for documenting your womb experiences, do a quick ritual to prepare the blank pages for your words...

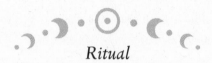

Ritual
Blessing Your Womb Journal

Place the journal in your lap and take some breaths, deep into your womb.

Place one hand over your journal and one hand over your womb as you continue to take your womb breaths. In doing this, you are establishing a deep connection between your womb and journal. This will help you feel safe to process and express, in written words, all the womb is experiencing.

Imagine that love is pouring from your heart, down your arm, through your palm, and into the journal. Visualize that love blessing your journal. Then, focus on the center of your heart, and say out loud or in your head, "May this Womb Journal bring love, healing, and transformation into my life."

When you're ready to write, you can record your first entry in your journal. As you do write, try to continue your womb breathing and stay connected to your body. This will support you in accessing deeper emotions and help you find your flow with the writing process.

CHAPTER 1 TAKEAWAYS

- Every woman's womb is a power source. It gives her the ability to heal her body, relationships, sex life, and emotions. It's a place where she can access her creative energy, increase feelings of pleasure, and spark a natural ease and joy within.

- Our wombs carry imprints of past hurts. If we haven't processed and released them from our bodies, they will stay there, until we're ready to deal with them.

- A woman's reproductive system is for much more than making babies. It's a place women can connect to in order to find creative power, joy, grounding, and rejuvenation.

- A Womb Journal is a great tool for capturing parts of your journey. Writing also works wonders for helping us heal, process, and understand what happens to us more deeply.

Chapter 2

WOMB BREATHING

"When you breathe in mindfully, you bring your mind home to your body."
—Thich Nhat Hanh[3]

During my first son's birth, there was a cry. I had heard him right away, the moment he was pulled from my womb. With my second son, there was silence. At first, I hadn't noticed it. I was too full of adrenaline. I had pushed him out naturally, with no epidural, something I wasn't entirely certain I could actually do.

But after hours of stops and starts, and many threats of a C-section from doctors along the way, I had done it. I had vaginally birthed my second child into the world.

Although my husband stood by my decision, some in my family had said it couldn't be done. Since my first one had been born by C-section, they assumed that my body wasn't equipped to handle a vaginal birth and that the second one would be born that way, too. It felt good to prove all of them wrong.

Except, after I pushed the baby out, I looked at my husband's face, and his expression was one of deep concern. That's when I realized: my baby hadn't taken his first breath, nor did he cry.

---

3. Thich Nhat Hahn, "The Way Out Is In," April 15, 2014, in *Thich Nhat Hanh Dharma Talks*, podcast, audio, 1:47.

Some of the hospital staff had carried him over to the resuscitation area. They were quiet, yet calm, like they had done this many times before. My husband and I both watched, not exchanging a single word between us. Then, within seconds, my baby took his first breath, and started to cry.

The entire room seemed to sigh with relief.

When a baby is born, that first breath is everything. It marks a pivotal moment of the baby's separation from the womb, where they must begin the lifelong process of breathing.

The average adult breathes twenty thousand breaths each and every day; but how many of those twenty thousand breaths are we actually conscious of? As an automatic function controlled by the medulla oblongata in the base of our brains, breathing is something that happens without any thought, intention, or action on our part.

Our body is wired with intelligence, working with us at all times, even as we're focused on a gazillion other details whirling around in our brains. Even when we're unconscious and in a deep state of slumber, our brains continue to operate, driving the breathing process along. Luckily for us, this involuntary function is always working to keep us breathing and, of course, *alive*.

While our body holds exponential brilliance and capacity, that doesn't mean we should shrug our shoulders and disconnect from our physical beings. Breathing is something that happens automatically, but when we can start to become more conscious of it, when we can work to deepen and enhance it, we can wake up our inherent abilities for self-healing and energy enhancement, while promoting a deep sense of mental health and well-being.

As babies and young children, we all used to breathe the way we were meant to, surrendering to each inhale and exhale as it came, allowing each part of the breath to be drawn out to fullness, with each inhale reaching all the way down into the diaphragm.

For adults, breathing becomes encumbered by all the stress, chaos, and responsibilities of our daily lives. Shallow breathing into the chest becomes the norm, and rarely do many of us stop to allow each inhale and exhale to reach its fullest potential. The more fast-paced our world has become, the more fast-paced our breaths have become. In this digital age where headlines in the media become obsolete seconds after they're published, many of us seem to be in perpetual search mode, monitoring our phones for new notifications or scrolling endlessly through our social media feeds for the next fix. This lifestyle has promoted a cycle of shallow and unhealthy breathing.

It's time to start embracing slow living, to turn back into ourselves, to the rhythm of our bodies, so we can play an intentional role in how we feel and show up in the world.

WHY IS BREATHING SO IMPORTANT?

Breathing is a wildly essential part of life, for obvious reasons. Without breathing, we wouldn't be able to take in the oxygen necessary to sustain our lives. Beyond that, breathing is also important for strengthening the immune system, healing, and supplying the brain cells with much-needed oxygen.

I truly believe that the quality of your life depends greatly upon the quality of your breathing. If you go for only shallow, quick, choppy breaths, your life will come out that way. You will feel disjointed in your mind and spirit; you'll feel a sharp disconnect from your body and the wisdom within it. On the other hand, if your breathing is slow, intentional, and deep, you will cultivate a rich vibrancy within your being. This rich vibrancy will color your life. It will bring depth, joy, energy, and balance to your every moment.

Slow, intentional, deep breathing is the first step toward accessing the gift that is your womb. If your breathing is rushed and shallow, you'll have a tough time trying to connect to your body and womb. But if you slow down and devote your attention toward intentionally working with your breath, something new and exhilarating will start to happen. You'll start to feel and experience your energy in a way that is unrestrained—that is much more expansive than you ever thought possible.

Your fullest breath will bring forth your fullest life.

The breath has the ability to activate your capacity for healing, energy, and wellness. Connecting to your breath will help you become more familiar with your womb in ways that aren't just limited to menstruation, pregnancy, or childbirth. Each and every womb is unique, just as each and every woman on the planet is unique. Your womb holds the imprint of your emotions, your experiences, your joys and pains. And although it will be unlike any other, it will still have access to the same power as others. Take control of your breath, and you can access this power much more quickly.

Our feelings and emotions have the power to change the rhythm, depth, and quality of our breathing.

Do you ever notice what happens when you get super nervous? As much as I love to be up in front of people, teaching a meditation class or leading a women's circle, I sometimes feel a ton of nervousness beforehand. Waves of nausea ripple through me, and I feel all the muscles in my body tighten. Along with all this, I also notice that my breathing becomes very shallow and choppy. I find myself audibly gasping for breaths, which only perpetuates the nervous, anxious cycle I've found myself in.

Without allowing my body a chance to relax by way of a slow, deep, intentional breath, I remain a bundle of nerves. Since I'm aware of all this—and I'm also aware of dozens of breathing techniques that can guide me through these moments—I try to slow down and bring myself back to my body and to calmness. And if I don't, that nervousness dissipates the second I'm up there, leading the class and speaking. All the buildup and anticipation impacts my breathing pattern in a dramatic way.

When we're angry, sad, scared, or confused, our breathing also goes through shifts; some more subtle than others, but it's always happening, even though we might not really pay it any mind.

A recent study revealed that our emotions do impact the way we breathe.[4] In the study, the breathing patterns of participants were observed as they went

---

4. Emma Seppälä, "Breathing: The Little Known Secret to Peace of Mind," *Psychology Today*, April 15, 2013, https://www.psychologytoday.com/us/blog/feeling-it/201304/breathing-the-little-known-secret-peace-mind.

through various emotions, like happiness, fear, or sadness. Researchers made notes of these various breathing patterns, and when a set of new participants came in, they were given the specific breathing patterns to emulate. The participants weren't told about the certain emotion associated with the breathing pattern they were taking on. However, after breathing the way they were instructed to breathe, the participants actually felt the exact emotions that corresponded to those same breathing patterns.

By controlling our breaths,
we can control the way we feel.

Armed with the knowledge that we can control the way we breathe puts us in charge of our emotions. If you're struggling with anger issues, crippling worry, or deep sadness in your life, your breath can bring you back to yourself. Those uncomfortable emotions can begin to evaporate by you simply taking control of and being more conscious of the way you breathe. Just because your body does it automatically doesn't mean it's under control. Your awareness is a necessary part of the process in coming back to yourself, in aligning to the intelligence in your body and womb.

In the yogic chakra system, the womb is the place that corresponds to our emotions. *Chakra* is a Sanskrit word that means "wheel" or "disk," and it refers to centers of energy in our bodies. References to chakras were found in an ancient Indian text known as the Vedas, which was written sometime between 1500 and 1200 BCE. Our chakras run from the base of our spines all the way to the top of our heads, and they each correspond to different nerves, glands, and organs. Chakras reflect different aspects of ourselves and our lives, and help us balance and heal.

Our wombs are located in the second chakra, which is the center of our creativity, emotions, and sexuality. Emotions and feelings that we haven't yet processed and moved out of the body live in our wombs. They can live in other parts of our bodies as well. For some of us, our emotions are uncomfortable and difficult to deal with, and so we decide not to deal, and we keep pressing on with our lives.

---

*Not dealing with an emotion doesn't mean
the emotion magically goes away.*

An emotion is held within the body, waiting for us, waiting for that opportunity when we will be ready to process and heal. Since the body is so intelligent and is always working with you, know that it wants to process out the things causing pain and discomfort. The body wants you to remember. The womb wants you to remember.

The frustrating thing is that there hasn't been a great deal of research on the womb that is unrelated to fetuses and pregnancy. Based on what research has been done, we know babies are able to sense their mother's psychological state while in the womb.[5]

I remember, during my first pregnancy, reading a book that strongly advised all moms to stay calm, cool, and collected for the entire nine months, or else we'd be hurting our babies even before they come out of the womb. I don't know about you, but nine months is a long time to stay in a Zen-like state, and to not let anything get you down. Especially during pregnancy. You're growing a whole person, from start to finish, inside your body. You're bound to feel stressed, sad, scared, and worried during some part of that process. There will be joy and happiness and crazy amounts of bliss, too, but there will also be low points. This is just a part of life that must be embraced.

The key is not to try to avoid the pain or the grief or the heartache. It's to allow yourself the opportunity of feeling it. Not to deny it or stuff it down somewhere inside of you, only to have it seep into your life at the most inconvenient moment. It's about owning every single one of your feelings and emotions. Letting it all wash over you, so you can feel it in its fullness... and then moving on from it.

---

5. Curt A. Sandman, Elysia Poggi Davis, and Laura M. Glynn, "Prescient Human Fetuses Thrive," *Psychological Science* 23, no.1 (January 2012): 93–100.

Controlling your breathing does not mean "don't feel this anymore" or "pretend like it never happened." It does not mean you are putting your head in the sand and acting cloyingly positive, no matter what's going on in your life. You're still feeling your emotions, but you're staying tethered to your core. By controlling your breath, you're giving yourself and your emotions an anchor, a foundation. Instead of spiraling out of control, your breath can bring you back to balance and allow your emotions and feelings to move through you in a healthy way.

BEING POSITIVE

A deep, slow, and nurturing breath should never be used as a way of brushing off emotions or forcing a facade of positivity. When a friend comes to us in desperation, full of tears and melancholy after a horrendous breakup, we might be tempted to try to lift her up with the words *be positive*. But when one is going through pain, heartache, depression, or grief, "be positive" serves as a hollow form of advice. It's not what anyone wants to hear. The problem isn't that they're not being positive enough. All of us have struggles and burdens we must carry in this life, and when we try to gloss over them, we do ourselves a disservice. We don't allow ourselves to fully feel our emotions, to give ourselves the opportunity to absorb, process, and understand what we're experiencing.

*Instead of forcing a positive front to the world,
give yourself permission to feel sad, disappointed,
afraid, worried, or doubtful.*

As you allow yourself to feel and express, find your breath. Let your breath be the soothing balm to your spirit in the midst of heart-crushing grief or sorrow. Find your breath, and find your center again. And from that place, let the emotions, let the feelings, be felt. And once they're felt, you can begin to process them in a healthy way, so that you can start to heal and move forward.

Shaking Off Negative Thoughts

Becoming conscious of your womb means you start unlocking the brilliance that is stirring within every cell of your body. And to unlock that, the mind must be still, soft, and quiet. The mind must do away with the conventional modes of thinking that often include endless cycles of thoughts that hurt you instead of heal you.

Connecting to your body and your womb in a state of deep awareness requires that you allow the mind to take a back seat. It requires that you trust and love who you are, that you believe you are worth more than the negative things you sometimes tell yourself in your mind.

If thinking negative thoughts about yourself is something you know you do, you're not alone. Many of us find ourselves cycling through negative thoughts. We get caught in these cycles where we continue deepening those grooves of negativity in our minds, and it can become difficult to stop.

We get so used to thinking these kinds of disempowering thoughts that they start to happen on autopilot. We're not even fully cognizant of the fact that we're doing it because we're just so used to it.

To become BFF with your womb, you've got to push beyond those negative thoughts. Because if you don't, those negative thoughts will define your life. They will color everything you see and experience, filling your days with a kind of heaviness that will prevent you from pressing forward.

Consciously breathing offers a way of shaking off any negative thoughts. The reason being, when you breathe, you come into the present moment. And thoughts cannot exist when the mind is wildly present. That feeling of aliveness that bubbles up within you simply cannot be there if you're just in a state of recycling endless thoughts.

The breath brings you back to this moment so that you can reach out and grab the here and now. Being in the moment means you're awake to what's happening in your body and your womb. This is the state in which time doesn't exist. In which you don't perceive any boundaries or obstacles in life. All that exists is the moment, and your deep state of being in the moment.

The next time you find yourself battling with a barrage of negative thoughts, remember to take a deep breath. See how that affects you, how that pulls you out of the fog of your mental chatter. How it reminds you of the things you've forgotten—the things that are sacred and truly worth focusing on.

Um ... How Exactly Do I Take a Deep Breath?

An amazing yogi taught me a very simple trick for deepening the breath and our connection to it. All it takes is awareness.

All you need to do is start noticing your breath, without trying to force it in any way. Just notice the way it moves in and out of your body. Allow yourself to tune out all your surroundings so that you can be fully present to what your breath is revealing to you in each moment. That's all it takes.

Once you become aware of the breath, your body starts naturally wanting to go deeper and slower. If you try this and find it isn't naturally happening for you, focus instead on just slowing everything down. If you rush the breath, even with the intention of going deep, you risk cutting it off too short. But if you start to consciously slow down, not rushing through a single moment, you can start to expand your lung capacity.

In James Nestor's book *Breath*, he shares a series of fascinating adventures and findings on the breath. One of the things he mentions is that, in order to take a full, deep breath that will enhance wellness in our bodies, we must devote a whole 5.5 seconds to the inhale, as well as 5.5 seconds to the exhale.[6] Doing this brings the body into equilibrium. Try doing this for an entire day, and see how you feel by the end of it.

Since the body might be used to taking quicker, more shallow breaths, you'll have to devote your consciousness to the breath in order to ensure that it's long and deep. It might be impossible to time out 5.5 seconds each and every time. 'Cause if you did that, how would you be able to focus on anything else? But long and deep is the key here. Start out by counting 5.5

---

6. James Nestor, *Breath* (New York: Riverhead Books, 2020), 83.

seconds for each part of the breath in your head, and then after a couple of minutes, let the count go, but maintain your deep breathing.

INTRODUCING THE WOMB BREATH

One technique that can support you in breathing deeply is to focus on taking a "womb breath." A womb breath offers a quick way of bringing you into the present moment and connecting you to your body. It's also very simple to do…

As you're inhaling, you're visualizing the breath reaching all the way down into the womb, as far as it can go, and then when you're exhaling, you're sending that breath from the womb, all the way up and out the body.

As you're taking in a womb breath and breathing deeply, you'll notice your belly pushing outward. And when you exhale, you should notice your belly pulling back in toward the spine. That's when you know you're breathing deeply and engaging those lower diaphragmatic muscles.

Although it isn't physically possible for a breath, no matter how deep it is, to make it all the way to the womb, it's the visualization that matters. Allowing your mind to envision the breath reaching that depth in your body helps you relax and expand the length of your breath. In reality, the breath can only go so far as the lower part of the diaphragm. When the belly is pressing out, it is due to the diaphragm pressing down on it and pushing it out.

However, just because the breath is only going so far as the diaphragm physically, don't underestimate the power the breath has on the body as a whole. A full, deep breath has the ability to impact your cells, blood, organs, lymph, life force energy, and muscles. Breathing deeply is a healing elixir, a medicine for revitalizing the mind, body, and spirit. It's time to start taking this ability we have to tap into our breaths and using it to change our lives.

Bringing our presence into everything we do—whether it's womb breathing, taking out the trash, or catching up with a friend on the phone—will instantly ground us and relax the nervous system.

Practice

Womb Breath

You can take a womb breath from any position you're in, whether it's sitting, standing, or lying down. The beauty about womb breathing is that you can do it anytime, anyplace. This is a foundational breath that you can consistently use to bring balance to your daily life.

For this practice, lie down on your back on either the floor or a bed.

Place both hands over the lower part of your belly and your womb space. Allow all your muscles to melt into the surface underneath you.

And now, through the nose, take a deep inhale. On your inhale, imagine you are sending the breath all the way down into your womb, underneath your hands. As you do so, feel the belly rise up, away from the spine.

As you exhale now, also through the nose, imagine you are moving that breath from the womb and all the way up and out the nostrils. Feel the belly pulling away from your hands and back in toward the spine.

Continue womb breathing for at least five minutes.

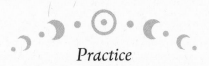

Practice

Extended Womb Breathing

You can either lie down or sit up for this one.

Place both hands over your lower belly and pelvis.

Inhale through the nose, and imagine you are guiding that breath all the way down into your womb.

Once you reach the end of that inhale, hold your breath. As you hold your breath, imagine that breath is massaging all your feminine parts—feel your womb, your ovaries, your fallopian tubes, your cervix, your vulva, and your vagina relaxing.

When you're ready to exhale, imagine you are drawing that breath out of the womb and back out of the body.

Repeat this breath for about five minutes.

This breathing practice is a great way of connecting to and establishing a deeper relationship with your precious reproductive organs. When you're concentrating your energy on nurturing this space through the breath, you will start to open up to the potential that is inherent there.

Simply by being quiet and directing your focus and breath to these parts of yourself, you can start to awaken your womb power. You can bring a vitality back to those parts of yourself that you might have been neglecting for a long time. As you do this exercise, your body will soften and surrender to the magic that is you.

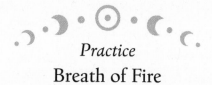

Practice

Breath of Fire

The breath of fire is a Kundalini Yoga practice that is used to energize, balance, and refresh the body. Kundalini Yoga is a practice that involves opening up your chakras as well as a potent kind of energy that exists at the base of the spine. This breathing practice involves pumping the belly out on the exhale rapidly, and it is really great for removing stuck or stagnant energy in your belly and womb.

To practice this breath, sit up nice and straight.

Now, take a normal inhale through the nose, and then quickly push the exhale out of the nose.

Continue doing this breath over and over. You should be able to hear the bursts of your exhale quickly being pushed out of your nose. Your stomach will also be pumping in and out as you do this.

Go slowly at first as you're getting the hang of it. When you feel comfortable, you can go faster.

Try to start out with a set of twenty of these rapid breaths. Then rest for a few seconds, and then do twenty more.

Avoid the breath of fire practice if you're pregnant or have heart conditions. Also, if your body doesn't feel comfortable doing this practice, ease off a bit and slow down. Listen to what your body needs, and go at a pace that works for you.

Practice
The 5.5 Breath

If you'd like to try getting more natural at doing a 5.5 inhale and 5.5 exhale throughout the day, start by actually counting while you're breathing.

Inhale through the nose, slowly and deeply, and count to 5.5 seconds in your head.

Now, start to exhale, and also count to 5.5 seconds in your head.

Continue doing this for a couple of minutes, until your lungs seem used to the 5.5-second count. Then you can let go of the count, but just continue breathing deeply and naturally here.

The idea isn't that you're going to nail 5.5 seconds exactly, but after you know what it feels like, you'll be able to approximate it.

Practice
HA Breath

Another great breath for cleansing the womb area is the HA breath.

Take a quick inhale, and on your exhale, push out the sound *HA*.

Do it quickly, without break, and just allow the HA to ease out of you.

You should feel your belly pushing out as well. This breathing practice will create energy in your body, clear your mind, and help push worry and negativity out of your system.

WOMB BREATHE WHILE YOU READ

As you read through the rest of this book, you might want to think about using the time to be conscious of your breathing. Practice womb breaths as you read, and they'll allow you to absorb the words in a deeper way. Being more mindful and conscious of your breathing automatically makes you more mindful and conscious of everything within and around you. So, take those womb breaths as often as you can—while you're in line at the grocery store, sitting at your desk, taking a shower, walking to the mailbox, making love. Womb breathing will transform the way you feel, think, move, and speak. Breathing this way will give you a glowing complexion, a more relaxed mind, and a tangible feeling of bliss running effortlessly through the body.

CHAPTER 2 TAKEAWAYS

- The quality of your life depends upon the quality of your breaths.
- The slower, deeper, and more intentional your breathing is, the more you can work to cleanse and activate the womb.
- By controlling your breath, you can find balance in your feelings and emotions.
- We must give ourselves permission to feel our emotions so that we can process and understand them.
- Womb breathing consistently is a powerful way of creating the foundation for an amazing day.

Chapter 3

YOUR WOMB STORY

"There is no greater agony than bearing an untold story inside you."
—*Zora Neale Hurston*[7]

In 2018, I almost died.

It was a few days after the Thanksgiving holiday, a little after 4:00 a.m. I was awoken from my sleep by a pain in my stomach unlike anything I had ever experienced. This wasn't your average stomachache. It felt like someone had dug a sharp blade into my stomach and was twisting it, deeper and deeper.

Within minutes, my husband and I were out the door. He drove me to the nearest emergency room while I screamed on the floor of the car, in too much pain to sit still.

When we got to the hospital, they tried various medications and doses to ease the pain, but it just wouldn't let up. Eventually they found that Dilaudid did the trick. Once they had me calm and able to lie still in my hospital bed, they were able to launch into a battery of tests to determine what the issue was. In the beginning, they suspected it might have been something like a kidney stone.

---

7. Zora Neale Hurston, *Dust Tracks on a Road* (New York: HarperCollins, 1996), 176.

After hours of tests, the doctor had finally discovered something on a CT scan. But he wasn't quite sure what he was looking at. The scan showed him something abnormal in my stomach. And I could tell by the expression on his face that this was serious. In a calm voice, he told me that it was necessary to rush into surgery.

Several hours later, after I awoke from the procedure, the doctor told me that when he opened me up, he found something that he had never, in his entire career, seen before. My small intestine had been tied in a tight knot. Literally tied, like a shoelace. It had been tied so tightly that the tissue of the intestine had already started to die out.

During surgery, the doctor had actually called in two other doctors. They all tried to untie the tight knot, but nothing was working. And since a good 60 percent of my intestine no longer contained living tissue, they would have to cut it all out anyway. And so they did, fusing the leftover 40 percent of my small intestine together and saving my life in the process.

The surgeon said that I was a mere six hours away from the tissue in my small intestine dying out completely. And if that had happened, there would've been nothing he could've done to save me.

Being suddenly so close to death was a very surreal experience. Since I've always been healthy and disciplined about taking care of my body, I had never in a million years imagined something like this could happen to me.

The culprit was the scar tissue in my abdomen, which happened as a result of the C-section I had with my firstborn. Whenever we're cut into, our bodies form scar tissue as a way of healing and protecting us. But with time, this scar tissue creates a web in the body, forming adhesions, which contain stickiness. This stickiness is what allowed for my small intestine to get caught and start twisting.

Although C-sections are performed at an alarmingly high rate in the United States and other countries in the world, no one is really educating women on the importance of breaking up and softening their scar tissue after surgery. Adhesions from the scars actually end up restricting the soft tissue. This can cause chronic pain, numbness, tingling, and tightness in the abdomen. It can also lead to bowel obstructions, where your small intestine gets stuck and twists, like it did to me. My case, with the knot, was a pretty severe version.

But it didn't end there. My life-saving surgery back in 2018 ended up creating more scar tissue and adhesions, which meant more opportunities for obstructions. Three years later, I ended up having several other small bowel obstructions, back-to-back. I ended up staying at the hospital for a total of fourteen days over three different visits.

A couple of the obstructions were resolved by a nasogastric tube that nurses stuck up my nose, down my throat, and into my stomach. This tube suctioned out my stomach, until eventually the twists resolved on their own. It's a painful and interminable process I don't ever want to relive. The tube basically stays inside of you for days straight. It hurts every time you swallow or talk, and you aren't able to eat or drink during the whole ordeal.

After that happened in early 2022, I decided that enough was enough. I was done listening to doctors who all told me that nothing could be done to break up my scar tissue, and that I would just have to experience these obstructions for the rest of my life. I started looking into solutions to heal my body, belly, and womb from what it experienced during my C-section. I found microcurrent therapy, myofascial release therapy, and a host of other things that have been helping me release my scar tissue and bring my womb and belly back into balance.

All these episodes have been the latest installments of my Womb Story. It's part of my womb's history, and although it has been a tough period in my life, it's grounding to reflect on it, to own it. It's all part of the healing process.

When I was pregnant with my firstborn, I was resolved. I knew I didn't want a C-section, and that it just wasn't the right path for me. I didn't want my womb cut. I wanted to deliver this baby naturally, with no meds. And so, I did everything I could to prepare for labor and delivery. I read books, exercised, went to classes, and even learned hypnotherapy techniques that supposedly worked to facilitate a natural birth.

None of that mattered in the end. After a series of issues, the baby just wouldn't come out, no matter how hard I pushed. The hospital staff was starting to get short and impatient with me. They showed me that the baby's heart rate was dropping on the monitor, and told me that a C-section had to happen *now*. I was crushed, but I accepted it, as I tried hard to fight back my tears. I didn't want the life of my precious baby to be at risk.

After the C-section, I remember feeling this numbness in my womb that lingered for weeks. Deep inside, I felt disappointed in myself, like my body wasn't good enough, like I hadn't been strong enough. I wondered if the hospital staff really thought my baby was in danger, or if they had just wanted to clear the room and get it all over with already. I also wondered if things would've been different if I had hired a doula.

I could've never imagined at that time, years later, that the C-section would have resulted in my being so close to death. I've spent many moments since then wondering about what could have been done to make things go differently.

But this is part of my story. It belongs to me. It's part of what makes me who I am now. And as challenging as things have been, I would not change who I am for anything in the world.

Our stories define us. They are interwoven with the fabric of who we are. Instead of pushing our own unique experiences aside, it's time to embrace them.

Embracing our stories helps us heal and evolve.

What is your Womb Story?

What has your womb experienced during this lifetime?

Many of us probably haven't considered these questions before. But it's time to start asking and reflecting. In order to own the power inherent in our wombs, we must recognize their histories. Knowing the history of the womb is the beginning of this new journey, the start to truly understanding who you are and where you've been. One of the most powerful ways to do this is through writing out your Womb Story.

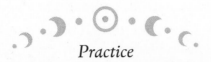

Practice

Writing Your Womb Story

Grab your Womb Journal, or a piece of paper, and something to write with.

Find a quiet place where you won't be disturbed during this time. Light a candle if you're able to.

Also, try to drink some water before you start journaling. At least fifteen to twenty ounces. Doing this will put you in a state of flow and begin to activate the womb area. The element that is connected to the womb is water, so drinking before your writing begins is an important part of this practice.

Once you're ready to start journaling, take a deep breath and write. Write about all your womb has been through so far. You can write about things like past sexual experiences, surgeries, childbirth, pregnancy, or any physical issues. You can also write about your connection to your womb. Have you been conscious of nurturing it and giving it your love and attention? Why or why not?

You can also focus on any struggles you've had with expressing your sensuality or navigating certain romantic relationships from your past, since all of that is tied into the womb as well. Also, since the womb holds on to emotions, you can even write about certain emotions you haven't been able to let go of or move on from in your life.

Let your Womb Story flow.

Remember, this is your story, and no one else's.

Feel the power that comes with owning your experiences. Feel the power that comes with knowing it is up to you to determine how to move forward from here. You, and only you, can shape what comes next.

When you're finished writing, take some womb breaths. Place both hands on your womb and read the words you've written. Take it all in. That's all you need to do. It isn't necessary to "fix" anything, or to justify why certain things happened the way they did. Just simply read and let your story be what it is.

Know that your Womb Story is far from over, and that there will be so much more to experience and write about in the days ahead.

CHAPTER 3 TAKEAWAYS

- Your Womb Story matters. It defines who you are and will help you understand the power you hold inside of you.
- Take time to reflect and write about your Womb Story. Let go of the need to "fix" certain aspects of your story. Make space for accepting and allowing your story to be what it is. Before you start writing your Womb Story, try to drink fifteen to twenty ounces of water. The water will put you in a state of flow and give you more access to your emotions. This will help you write more freely.

Chapter 4

LISTEN TO
YOUR WOMB

"When the womb is honored and respected, she becomes a channel of power, creativity, and beauty—and joy reigns on earth. When her voice goes unheard, unanswered, denied, the womb becomes a vessel of disease."

—Queen Afua[8]

For the past decade, a growing number of women have chosen not to have children. The birthrate here in the United States has declined by nearly 20 percent from 2007 to 2020.[9] And yet this continues to be looked at as taboo, as if women who make this choice have something severely wrong with them.

A recent study revealed that the womb may play a role in brain function and memory.[10] As we continue to understand more about the womb, people will hopefully begin to realize that wombs are for more than just developing fetuses and popping out babies. Wombs are sources of great potential, intelligence, and healing—and so are the women who carry them.

When you think about it, it's kind of rebellious to connect to your womb at a deeper level and to notice it in ways that go beyond pregnancy. Doing this is outside the norm. It's not the average path society expects you to take.

---

8. Queen Afua, *Sacred Woman* (New York: One World, 2000), 2.

9. Melissa S. Kearney and Phillip Levine, "Will births in the US rebound? Probably not." The Brookings Institution, May 24, 2021, https://www.brookings.edu/blog/up-front/2021/05/24/will-births-in-the-us-rebound-probably-not/.

10. Stephanie V. Koebele et al., "Hysterectomy Uniquely Impacts Spatial Memory in a Rat Model: A Role for the Nonpregnant Uterus in Cognitive Processes," *Endocrinology* 160, no. 1 (January 2019): 1–19.

*By forging a relationship with your womb, you're
taking your power back. You're taking ownership of your
body, which is one of the most empowering gifts you
can give yourself as a woman.*

With misogynistic attitudes and structures pervading our culture, it can be difficult to trust oneself and stay connected to who we really are. This is why cultivating an awareness of the womb is so essential. It's the way we find ourselves again. Using the womb as an anchor, we can always find our way back to the body, to loving and cherishing who we are.

One of the ways we can start waking up to the wild power present in the womb is simply by listening to it. When we start listening to our wombs, the energies of wisdom and intuition begin to blossom within. Now, listening might sound like a hard thing to do at first, but once you start doing it, it becomes a simple, pleasurable practice. In fact, it goes beyond even being a practice. It just becomes a part of who you are and what you naturally do.

When you awaken this natural instinct to really hear what your womb is telling you, you become an unstoppable force.

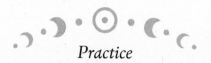

Practice
Listening to Your Womb

Your uterus is thrumming with intelligence, and you can tap into it anytime you need wisdom, guidance, or support. To do this listening practice, carve out at least five to ten minutes to hear the messages your womb has to share with you.

Place both hands over your womb, below the navel.

Close your eyes and take a few womb breaths. Remember to go slowly here, moving the breath in and out, seeing each inhale and exhale all the way to the end.

Next, ask your womb (mentally or out loud), *What do you want to tell me?*

Once you've asked the question, go back to taking deep womb breaths as you listen for an answer.

The answer might come as a quiet voice from deep within. It might come as a sensation fluttering inside your chest. It might be a sudden vision that comes into your mind from out of nowhere. Don't force anything. Just let the answer be what it wants to be.

And don't get frustrated if you try this and can't really "hear" anything at first. As you are starting to connect with the womb, it might be choppy in the beginning. But if you make time to consistently listen to your womb, you'll start to develop an understanding of how to connect more deeply and understand the answer that's being given to you.

Do You Hear That?

The body houses deep intelligence within. Between all the organs, the blood, the lymph, the muscles, and the tissues, there is an innate synchronization that is working around the clock to keep your body functioning. This is something we take for granted, since it all happens automatically, without any direction from us.

Our body as a whole is always in communication with us. We just have to become more conscious of it to be able to hear and understand what it wants to tell us. Oftentimes we actually do hear our bodies loud and clear, but it's a narrative that doesn't suit our needs at the moment. So, we shrug it all off and move on with our lives.

This might sound familiar to you. You might hear that voice within telling you to stop, to slow down, to cease with pushing yourself any further. But then you do it anyway. You destroy yourself by overworking, or getting a few hours of sleep a night, or saying yes to something you really wanted to say no to.

Women: we've got to stop ignoring those feelings, those voices calling to us from within. We've got to start the practice of listening deeply to our wombs and bodies so we know exactly what we need at all times. When we listen, we start to shake the dust off our own internal compass. And when that happens, we're able to show up, create, speak, love, and make an impact in ways we never imagined were possible.

Listening to the body is an act of self-love.

Why don't we listen to ourselves enough?

Instead of following our inner wisdom, we're grappling around outside of ourselves to search for meaning and fulfillment. Those things can never be found on the outside, yet the world tells us otherwise. It prides itself upon external markers of success and achievement.

Our systems aren't set up in ways that truly nourish and empower the whole being. Our schools are filling children's minds with facts, but what is being done to support their bodies and hearts? Our gigantic corporations are all for expanding the bottom line, but what about really nurturing, recognizing, and actively supporting the evolution of each worker who is part of the process? This is the world the people before us helped create, the world all of us alive today continue to perpetuate.

Our world is built on logic and reason. The mind is prized above all else. Many of us have internalized this idea, allowing our minds to lead the way. So much so that we've lost that beautiful and innate connection to the wisdom available in the womb, the heart, and the body as a whole. The mind is such a small percentage of who you really are. Obviously, we all need our minds and brains, but we need to bring in the rest of ourselves, too. The mind is a pro when it comes to analyzing and thinking things through. But bring the womb into the equation, and you've got a fireball of intuition and power on your side. Throw the heart into the equation as well—*and now we're talking*.

I used to be the worst at making decisions. I'd weigh the pros and cons of this and that. Sometimes I'd even grab a piece of paper and write everything out so I could see it all clearly. I just didn't want to make the wrong choice.

If you struggle to make decisions, have an overactive mind, or deal with worry and self-doubt, listening to your womb and body will help tremendously. It will bring more clarity and flow inside your body and mind.

When you start listening to your womb and your body, you don't have to worry about making the wrong choice. You feel the answer deep inside of you, and you *just know* which way to go.

If your mind isn't clear, it means you're spending too much time in your head and not enough time in your body.

The temple of your body is a sacred space, a miracle that is yours to bless and nurture each and every day. Just by listening to it, you can walk the direct path to deep, sustainable joy, sensuality, purpose, and transformation. By starting with the womb, your power source, you can begin to hone in on all the feelings and emotions within, to align to the feminine wisdom that's just waiting to be unleashed.

All it takes is to get quiet and listen. To let all the distractions fall away, so that you can be present to what's available now, in this moment. When you listen, you can truly start to awaken your inner power and intuition.

CHAPTER 4 TAKEAWAYS

- Your womb carries wisdom and intelligence. Take time to listen to it, and you will develop your intuition and connection to the body.
- An overactive mind can indicate you aren't connected to your body. To banish the chatter, worry, and self-doubt, just tune in and let the womb be heard.

Chapter 5

TALK TO YOUR WOMB

"Language creates reality. Words have power. Speak always to create joy."
—*Deepak Chopra*[11]

For many years, I wanted to write a book. I never really knew what it would be about, just that I wanted to write it. This feeling was always with me. But I often found myself trying to quiet it. I'd tell myself that it was simply foolish, because honestly, what would *I* write about? What did I have of value to put down on paper and share with the world?

After years of these disempowering thoughts zipping through my mind, keeping me in my place and not giving me the power to take action on what was in my heart, I realized I was only hurting myself. I knew that these thoughts were keeping me from actualizing my potential and doing what I wanted to do with my life.

So, one day, I started writing. And within six months, I had a draft of my first book: *Fierce Woman: Wake Up Your Badass Self.*

If I had continued to think those same thoughts, I wouldn't be sitting here right now, writing my second book. I would've still been caught in a situation where my heart was feeling one thing, yet my mind, out of fear,

---

11. Deepak Chopra, Facebook, December 9, 2011, https://www.facebook.com/DeepakChopra/posts/language-creates-reality-words-have-power-speak-always-to-create-joy/10150435500685665/.

was allowing me to believe and keep in line with another reality that simply did not serve me.

Our thoughts carry a great deal of magnetic energy. What we think creates the foundation for what we see, experience, and feel in our day-to-day lives. Thoughts don't merely live in their compartment in the mind, unable to affect or penetrate any other aspect of our lives. Thoughts set the tone. They can inspire and propel us forward, toward all that we think we're worthy of; or, they can weigh us down, and make us feel like we're carrying a bag of bricks on our backs with every step we take.

Since our wombs are able to absorb all our feelings and emotions, they're also impacted by the kinds of thoughts we think. The more uplifting our thoughts are, the more womb wellness we'll be able to cultivate. This is because thoughts lead to feelings and emotions. Someone who is constantly thinking that their life has no meaning or purpose will start to cultivate feelings based on those thoughts. They might feel depressed, angry, or fearful, flooding the heart and womb with a dense kind of negative energy.

When these kinds of feelings and emotions are propelled to live in our bodies based on these negative thought patterns, we must try to process what we're experiencing and move on. Stopping the cycle of negative thoughts and starting to replace them with kinder ones is essential.

Thinking kind thoughts about yourself might not come easy to some of us. If you're used to letting your mind run rampant with thoughts that cut down the beauty of what you are, the idea of thinking positively about yourself might sound like an unattainable, faraway goal to you. But it doesn't have to be.

Cultivating kind thoughts about oneself forges the path toward a life of joy and purpose.

Treating ourselves kindly begins with cultivating more positive, empowering thoughts about ourselves. If we can start thinking better about ourselves, we will automatically start to take care of ourselves more. We will love and cherish ourselves more, which will, in turn, have an impact on everything we do in the world. Kinder thoughts will inspire us to shine brighter and be who we are, unapologetically.

Our thoughts are in our control. No one else can do the work of thinking kinder thoughts for us, but ourselves. It might be tough, especially if you're used to playing out the same old, unhelpful thought patterns about yourself; but don't let that deter you. You can nurture empowering thoughts that will amplify the power in your womb and infuse your days with a new kind of potential. Make a commitment to nurture kind and loving thoughts, and watch your life expand.

AFFIRMATIONS

One of the most powerful ways to transform the mind is to use positive affirmations. By affirming something in the positive, as if it's happening in this moment, we can set the stage for more confident and empowered feelings to flow through us.

You've probably already heard a great deal about the power of affirmations. This is nothing new and revolutionary. Sometimes the mind just needs a simple way of clearing itself and aligning back to its potential. If you notice the negative thought cycle starting to spin in your mind, you can create one affirmation that will bring you back to the present moment and shut down all that disempowered thinking.

Make your sentence something that's easy to say and remember. It should be short and to the point. Something like, *I am amazing.* Or, *I am a blessing.*

Affirmations must be stated in the present tense, as if they're happening in the moment. Think these words in your head or say them out loud. Whatever the affirmation is, make sure the words are kind, and that they confirm and acknowledge the powerhouse of a woman you truly are.

WOMBFIRMATIONS

Making affirmations directly to the womb is a great way of showering that part of yourself with love and attention.

How often do we say loving words about our bodies? How often do we look into the mirror and truly admire what we see?

A wombfirmation is a way of speaking nurturing words directly to your womb. Since your womb is your internal power source, sending it some love via wombfirmation will help amplify and enhance your magic even more.

Imagine a world where women's bodies are celebrated with reverence and love instead of objectified. Imagine standing in a new culture, where our bodies are given the respect and admiration they deserve, instead of being hurt, shamed, or abused.

We cannot control the world around us. Heck, we can't even control the people who populate our own lives, as tempting as it may be to try to change them sometimes. But we can control how we show up every day. We can make sure our thoughts are vibrating at the highest level so that our potential, the full extent of our love and creative power, is radiantly expressed on this planet. We can love and honor our bodies, despite centuries of the patriarchal order of things attempting to dictate to us that we're not good enough.

Placing your hands over your womb and making a wombfirmation is a step in that direction. Show love toward your womb, and it will show love right back to you.

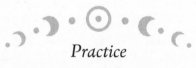

Practice
Using Wombfirmations

Find a quiet place to sit. Place your hands gently over your womb and take a few womb breaths here.

Now, take some time to speak affirmations to your womb. You can state one affirmation over and over again. Or you can speak a set of different affirmations. Whatever feels best to you is the right way to go about this practice.

Here are some wombfirmation examples you might want to use:

- I love and honor my womb.
- My womb is powerful.
- With my womb, I can create anything I want.

- My womb is overflowing with abundance.
- My womb is a place of joy and love.
- I am a Womb Goddess.
- I am grateful for my womb.
- My womb is sacred and divine.
- My womb is connected to all wombs.
- My womb is beautiful.
- My womb is blessed.
- My womb is a blessing.

Use these wombfirmations to bring a deeper state of ease and joy into your body. At first, it might be difficult for you to say some of these phrases. You might feel disconnected from them; you might feel the words you're saying are simply untrue. Push through those feelings and allow yourself to relax into your womb.

By simply relaxing into your womb, you clear the path ahead and allow your mind to release its grip of control.

CHAPTER 5 TAKEAWAYS

- Our thoughts carry great energy and set the foundation for our day-to-day lives.
- Disempowering thoughts will bring about experiences and situations that are in like vibration.
- Think kind thoughts about yourself, and you will allow your potential to unfurl.
- Our wombs are impacted by the thoughts we think.
- Use the powerful practice of wombfirmation to speak kindness and send love to your womb. Speaking kind words about your womb can deeply transform your life.

Chapter 6

TOUCH YOUR WOMB

"Touch seems to be as essential as sunlight."
    —Diane Ackerman[12]

For the longest time, I was afraid to look at my belly.

After the emergency surgery where my belly had to be cut open in 2018, the changes were severe.

To be honest, my belly had changed significantly even before that, after the births of both my children. The smooth, flat belly I used to have as a young woman was no longer. And this wasn't something I embraced right away.

In fact, after my pregnancies, I patiently waited for things to change. I did my crunches to tone what I had lost. I bought all sorts of luxurious oils and creams that claimed they worked wonders on stretch marks and post-pregnancy bellies. I felt disappointed in myself, like somehow my body wasn't strong enough to remain untouched by the hand of pregnancy.

When my emergency surgery happened, just four years after my second pregnancy, there was no more time to pretend. I had to start accepting the changes that had occurred to my body. The cut on my belly was about four inches long, slicing all the way through the middle of my belly button. When I first laid eyes on it, I knew no amount of cream or oil in the world would put things back the way they were.

---

12. Diane Ackerman, *A Natural History of the Senses* (New York: Vintage, 1991), 80.

I spent months doing everything I could to not look at my belly. For someone who was so connected to and in love with her body, this was something different. I felt a disconnect—not just with my body, but with my whole way of being. It was as if a light had turned off within me.

Then one day, I realized I had to come back to myself. So, I started slow. At first, I wouldn't look at my belly directly; I'd just pull up my shirt and peek in the mirror for a few seconds. Then I'd extend that by a few more seconds the next time.

Soon I was able to start looking directly at my belly. It wasn't so bad, I realized. It wasn't perfect, but it wasn't so bad. I started to massage my belly, to send love through my hands to the parts of myself that had been forever changed. I wanted my body to know what it still meant to me. That I was still here. That I was starting to accept and love all of myself again.

It was a process (and still is). But I was able to start appreciating my belly again, to start honoring and cherishing it for all it has been through in this lifetime.

When we give our bodies the gift of our touch, we are claiming our power as women. The feminine energies inherent within us become tangible, heightening our creative output and bringing a certain kind of vibrancy into the body.

SELF-TOUCH

How often do you touch yourself?

How often do you touch your womb?

How often do you place your hands over your heart to check in on how you're feeling?

How often do you take your time to slather your body in intoxicating oils as you breathe deeply and allow yourself to surrender to the sensation on your skin?

And if you are doing these things, are you doing them every day?

Self-touch is a healing, rejuvenating way of connecting with the body. It's a way of honoring the body with your love and attention.

We're not touching ourselves nearly as much as we should be. Studies show that receiving touch from another person has the ability to create mental well-being, build trust, boost immunity, and soothe the nervous system.[13]

But what about self-touch? This is something no one ever really talks about. There is tremendous power that comes with the simple act of placing your hands on yourself. Our bodies actually crave touch each and every day.

When we make time for self-touch, we can open our bodies up to more presence, pleasure, and energy.

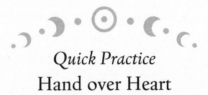

Quick Practice
Hand over Heart

Place your left hand over your heart with some nice firm pressure. Take a couple of belly breaths. And just notice your heart as you do this.

When you're finished, tune in and see how you feel. Do you notice the shift? Are you calmer and more relaxed? Do you feel any new kinds of sensations within?

SHOW YOUR BODY LOVE

As you go through this book, be sure to check in with yourself throughout. Notice how you're feeling during certain points and how those feelings inside of you might have changed based upon what you're reading or what practice you're trying out. If you notice a certain feeling or sensation coming up in your body, simply place a hand over it. Give it your attention and your touch, and notice what happens as a result.

For anyone who wants to love their body more deeply and unapologetically, self-touch is a positive action you can take immediately. It's something you can do right this second or any other time in your day.

---

13. Dacher Keltner, "Hands On Research: The Science of Touch," *Greater Good Magazine*, September 29, 2010, https://greatergood.berkeley.edu/article/item/hands_on_research.

> *Self-touch rewires the brain to start associating*
> *positive thoughts and feelings toward the body.*

Just start with a simple touch. You can place your hands over the top of your head and just breathe, feeling what's present there for you. You can stroke your arms and legs as a way of coming back to the present moment. You can put your hands over your womb and feel the magnificent power you contain within.

When you touch yourself, make sure you're present to that touch. Give yourself a moment to really breathe in and feel the touch. If you're not available and present to it, you won't get the benefits of the full healing experience.

Self-touch is an action you take, a way of showing you love and cherish who you are. It's a way of showing gratitude to your body, mind, heart, and spirit. If you're someone who struggles with fully accepting your body, self-touch can be your guide, bringing you back to the power of what you are.

For the purposes of this chapter, the self-touch we're exploring is non-sexual. It has nothing to do with self-pleasuring or masturbation. It is simply about allowing yourself to use touch as a way of connecting to the body, to healing, and to soothing the self.

SELF-TOUCH PRACTICES

Use these deeper self-touch practices to bathe yourself in healing, rejuvenating energies. Let yourself surrender to the comforting warmth of your own touch. You literally hold so much power in your hands.

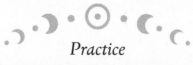

Practice
Head-to-Toe Touch

This practice may seem simple on the outside, but on the inside, it's coursing with power.

Get into a comfortable seated position, whether it's in a chair or on the floor.

Take a few deep womb breaths.

Start out by bringing both hands to the top of the head. Take a womb breath here as you feel your touch on the top of the head.

Next, place both palms over your eyes. Take another womb breath here.

Place both hands over your temples. Take a womb breath here.

Place both hands gently around the neck. Another womb breath here.

Continue this same practice as you move down the entire body. Stop and hold your chest, rib cage, belly, pelvis, thighs, knees, calves, and, finally, the feet.

At the end, wrap your arms around yourself in a big hug.

Make sure you complete one full womb breath at each area of the body you are holding on to.

If you'd like to devote more time to this practice, you can do two to three womb breaths per area.

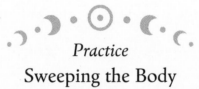

Practice
Sweeping the Body

This sweeping practice is a great way of ridding your body of any energy you don't want while tapping into your natural vibrancy. I love to do this sweeping practice first thing in the morning, or throughout the day, whenever I need to recharge my energy.

You can also do it whenever you've had an encounter or a conversation that makes you feel icky. We don't need to take on other people's stuff. But it's what we do unconsciously as we go about our days. We take on other people's energy, and it weighs us down. We make the mistake of thinking it's our own energy, and this brings us down even more, creating a feeling of helplessness, of not being able to get out from under all of it.

But the good news is that it just takes some awareness. As we stay aware and on top of what energy is coming toward us each day, and how we're feeling about it, we can take actions to move that energy on out before it becomes a major problem.

This sweeping practice is a way of doing that, and it just takes a minute or less.

First, stand up and take a deep womb breath.

Next, take both hands to the top of the head and brush energy off the head and out of the body, with the hands moving in a downward direction. Do this a few times. It's almost like you're brushing dust or lint off something. For example, let's say you see a whole mess of lint on your favorite coat. And so, you take a hand and brush down the coat to get it all off. That's basically the motion you're using for this sweeping exercise. You always want to sweep or brush away from the body, and in a downward motion.

After you're finished with the top of the head, proceed to go down the body and do this the whole way down. Brush down the sides of your head and face and out the body. Brush each area at least two to three times.

Brush down your neck and chest and out the body. Do one arm at a time.

When you get down to the womb, pay extra attention to this area. Be gentle as you brush down the womb and allow all that stuck energy to leave your body.

Finally, you can brush down your legs and feet and throw all that energy away, down into the earth beneath you.

Touching your body by doing the sweep practice feels awesome. And it's a great way of activating your cells and clearing your lymph of toxins.

Massage
Womb Self-Massage

Pay your womb some extra-special attention with a nice, gentle womb massage. For this one, grab a massage oil. You can even use olive, sesame, almond, or jojoba oil.

Lie on your back, and, as always, take a few womb breaths to center and relax yourself.

Put some oil on your belly and start to gently massage it.

Make circles across your belly with fingers from both hands. Be sure to keep breathing deeply as you do this. You can also use long strokes.

Next, start with the right hand, and take it across your body to the left side of your belly. With a little pressure, glide your hand across your belly, until you're all the way to the right side. Continue doing this a few more times with the right hand, until you've covered the entire belly.

Then switch sides. Take your left hand and bring it over to the right side of your belly. Press your fingers into your belly and wipe the hand all the way across until it comes back to the left side. Continue this here a few times.

Now, use your own instincts to stroke and massage your womb and belly area. You might notice that some parts need more attention than others. Be conscious and intentional during the massage, and don't forget to breathe.

With any kind of massage or self-touch you do, make sure to use all your senses. Stay present to the sensations within as you have your hands on yourself. Stay present to the breath. This will take your self-touch practice to a whole other level.

Healing Hack
Castor Oil Therapy

Castor oil is one of my go-to healing hacks. The kinds of benefits that castor oil provides to the womb are simply off the charts.

Castor oil gets the circulatory system going, which provides nourishment for all the organs in your reproductive and digestive systems. This oil reduces inflammation, eases menstrual cramps, balances hormones, improves bowel movements, and boosts fertility. You can use a castor oil pack on your lower belly and womb to receive all the amazing benefits.

To make one, you'll need the following items:

- Towel
- A piece of old flannel (long enough to wrap around your belly)
- Castor oil

And here's my quick-and-easy way of creating a castor oil pack without all the mess and hassle:

1. Place a long towel underneath you and lie down on it.
2. Put about a tablespoon of castor oil—more or less, depending upon your preference—in your hands, then massage it all into your lower belly and womb area.
3. Tie the flannel around your belly to cover up the oil and allow it a chance to more deeply penetrate the skin.
4. Put a heating pad or hot water bottle on top.

Once you've got your castor oil pack all set up, you can lie down and take it easy. I recommend leaving the pack on for at least an hour. You can even wear it overnight to soak up some extra healing benefits.

If you look online, most places will tell you to saturate your flannel in the oil, place that on your belly, and then wrap yourself in plastic wrap, like you're a chunk of leftover cheese. The thing is, castor oil can be extremely messy and runny, and it has a way of staining whatever it comes into contact with. So saturating flannel in oil seems stressful to me, which is why I recommend simply slathering some over your belly. And the idea of wrapping myself in plastic wrap doesn't exactly bring relaxing vibes to mind; not to mention, it isn't very environmentally friendly! Stick with my method, and you'll still reap the benefits. Just be sure not to use castor oil packs while you're pregnant, breastfeeding, or menstruating.

If you'd rather not DIY, check out Etsy.com for some nicely made castor oil packs. The premade ones ensure things are less messy, and it's a lot easier to get everything set up.

Since castor oil provides so many benefits, I use it all the time. Sometimes I just rub the stuff on my belly at the beginning of the day. Other times, I massage my belly with castor oil and go lie down in my infrared sauna to let the heat work its extra magic. I've even used it as a face mask and to cleanse and moisturize my skin in general.

Whatever you do, just grab a bottle of castor oil quick.

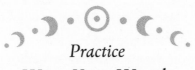

Practice

Wrap Your Womb

Wrapping your womb is a simple yet highly effective way of providing your womb with warmth, love, and healing. Known as a belly warmer, haramaki, womb wrap, or belly wrap, this item can bring about all kinds of benefits for your womb and body.

Womb wrapping brings stability and balance back to your womb and pelvic area. By holding everything snugly in place, it provides support and comfort. Also, as women, we sometimes tend to hold our stomachs in to give the appearance that we're thinner than we really are. This puts strain on our belly, womb, and pelvic region and separates us from the inner power we hold there. With the womb wrap on, you're able to just let your belly be, without tensing or holding it in. The wrap feels so comforting that the womb and belly just kind of relax into it.

Another benefit of wrapping the womb is the boost in circulation to that area of the body. This boost is healing for both your digestive and your reproductive organs.

In Eastern medicine, it's believed that the kidneys must stay warm in the body in order to ensure optimal health and immunity. Since the wrap also goes around the kidneys, it promotes warmth in that area and gives you a boost of immunity.

How To: Wrap the Womb

To wrap the womb, you don't need anything fancy. You can use a shawl or a scarf or any other kind of long fabric you might have. All you have to do is wrap it around your lower back and across your lower belly and tie it in a knot so that it stays. There are even some awesome Etsy creators who sell their own unique wraps, if you'd prefer to use something else. Just look up the words *belly warmer, stomach warmer, womb wrap,* or *haramaki.* This will give you a sense of the different options out there. They make them really stylish, too, so you can even wear them out in public.

You can wear your wrap for as long as you like. I will sometimes wear mine for a couple of hours, or even all day, if I want to show my womb some extra love and healing. I might take off my wrap if I'm working out or going to bed, but other than that, I can wear it while I'm doing just about anything. I love womb wrapping because not only is it a simple thing you can do whenever you feel like it, but it just feels really good. It's almost like a warm, comforting hug wrapping itself around your womb.

When I'm having menstrual cramps, wrapping my womb is instantly soothing. If you're using fabric, be careful not to wrap too tightly, though. You don't want to mess with your natural flow; just a light wrapping of your fabric will do the trick. If you've got a hara-maki or any other belly warmer, you can use that as well and not worry about it being too tight.

You can even wear your wrap or haramaki to bed to promote a restful night's sleep. I used to always take mine off before going to bed, but sometimes I keep mine on at night, too. I do notice I tend to feel more relaxed and fall asleep quicker when it's on.

Whether or not you wear your wrap or haramaki over or under your clothes is up to you. Many of these wraps and haramakis are made stylishly, with an array of different colors to choose from; so, you can feel confident and make a fashion statement while protecting your womb at the same time! When I wrap with a piece of fabric or a shawl, it can look a little awkward, so I only wear it that way when I'm inside the house. Find what works for you, and make it happen.

Wombs and pelvises can be very vulnerable areas on a woman's body. This is not to say that they're weak or inferior in any way. It just means that they hold a lot of energetic information and potential, and they are always working to maintain your inner feminine system. Wrapping these parts of yourself provides them not only with nurturing, but with protection. By protecting these sacred parts of your beautiful self, you are strengthening them and giving them an opportunity to recharge and rejuvenate when they need to. Although this isn't technically a form of you physically touching yourself, the wrap offers that sense of touch and stability that is deeply nurturing.

There are no rigid rules for wrapping your womb. Do it whenever you feel you need to, or do it daily to envelop your womb with super nurturing care and attention.

Chapter 6 Takeaways

- Self-touch is a way of honoring and celebrating your body.
- Our bodies want to feel balanced, cherished, healed, and accepted. This is why our bodies crave touch and nurturing each and every day.
- Touching the self has the power to rewire the brain and associate positive feelings toward our bodies.
- Use the breath and the senses to stay present and to allow yourself to truly receive all the benefits of self-touch and massage.
- Castor oil works absolute wonders for supporting the reproductive and digestive organs.
- Wrapping your belly and womb promotes a deep feeling of "receiving a big hug" around this area of your body. Do it for protection, healing, and strengthening of your feminine system.

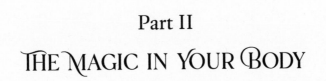

Part II

THE MAGIC IN YOUR BODY

Chapter 7

BREASTS

"Love and accept your breasts as they are. Breathe through the tiny holes in your nipples. Breathe into your heart center. Blossom a deep red rose. Spread its fragrance of beauty and goodness through the breasts. Smile down and feel the breasts glowing with warmth."

—*Minke de Vos*[14]

> NOTE: If you don't have physical breasts, you can still take part in all the practices in this chapter. The energy is still there, present in your chest and heart center. In practices where it says to "massage" or "meditate on" the breasts, use the chest area as your focus instead. And be sure to go from within the chest, and not merely on the surface of the chest. The idea is that you're activating your inner energy.

In 2019, I went on a book-signing tour for my first book, traveling to different locations throughout the United States. During the signings, I'd also give workshops where women would have an opportunity to experience some of the practices in the book.

Oftentimes, I'd be sharing some of the practices related to the breasts, and women would experience all kinds of emotions. Some women would cry; others would get really quiet and introspective. Many of them would say that they'd never held or connected to their breasts in that way before.

This is, in large part, due to the way our society currently focuses on breasts.

---

14. Minke de Vos, *Tao Tantric Arts for Women* (Vermont: Destiny Books, 2016), 159.

If you look at all the articles, books, and studies out there that involve our breasts, you'll find that the vast majority of them are written about breast cancer. In 2020, the International Agency for Research on Cancer, which is part of the World Health Organization, announced via press release that breast cancer had become the most prevalent form of cancer globally, making up 11.7 percent of new worldwide cancer cases.[15]

Knowing this, it's essential for women to be mindful about making healthy choices, paying attention to changes in the breasts, and getting screenings. Invasive breast cancer is a real issue, and one in eight women in the United States will develop it during her lifetime.[16]

Since there's no shortage of information out there on breast cancer, I truly feel it's time to start arming women with a deeper understanding of the power they carry in their breasts. One that isn't just based in breast cancer. Focusing on our breasts in this way is healthy to do, if it's part of a larger whole. That larger whole has to be about first initiating a deeper relationship and understanding of the beauty and energy we hold in our breasts.

Aside from breast cancer, the other two focuses on our breasts have to do with breastfeeding to give nourishment to a baby, or using the breasts to please and excite a romantic partner. There's nothing wrong with either of these things, obviously, but when they exist to the exclusion of the deeper meaning and potential carried in the breasts, we've got some serious problems. It's as if the pleasure and potential available in the breasts are for everyone but *ourselves*.

As women, we often mistake our power as being in our ability to give. We give our hearts, our bodies, our minds, our energy, our time, and, in some cases, our money. Sometimes we continue giving to people who aren't worthy of our time or attention. But we do it anyway, because we feel it's the right thing to do. It's in our feminine nature to carry this nurturing, giving, loving,

15. "Latest global cancer data: Cancer burden rises to 19.3 million new cases and 10.0 million cancer deaths in 2020," International Agency for Research on Cancer, December 15, 2020, https://www.iarc.who.int/wp-content/uploads/2020/12/pr292_E.pdf.

16. "Key Statistics for Breast Cancer," American Cancer Society, last modified January 12, 2022, https://www.cancer.org/cancer/breast-cancer/about/how-common-is-breast-cancer.html.

mama-like quality and to want to share that with the world. Giving just seems to be something embedded deep within our DNA.

Some of us see our worth as our ability to give. But this couldn't be further from the truth. Giving until the point of complete and utter depletion isn't going to make you worthy. You are already worthy, just as you are.

One of the most important qualities often used to describe the feminine is receptivity. That means we're receptive, able to receive what comes to us. If we truly want to unlock our gifts as women, we must learn the art of receiving. And we must receive as good as we give. That way, we're honoring ourselves and affirming our worth, while allowing for the cycle of giving and receiving to flow from us and to us.

Instead of feeling fear or anxiety surrounding the possibilities of being diagnosed with breast cancer, instead of looking at the breasts from the frame of giving nourishment or pleasure to another, it's time to start owning our breasts and the magic that exists within them. Once you start aligning to the energy and power of the breasts, you can use that alignment to connect to the energy present inside the womb space.

THE POWER INSIDE THE BREASTS

Within your beautiful breasts, you carry the potential for pleasure, healing, love, immunity, and power. When you can attune your focus and energy toward your breasts, you can access your superpowers and open the door to a juicier, more activated and passionate way of life. Since we've been distracted into only thinking of our breasts in certain limiting ways, we haven't really been able to experience the possibilities that lie in the breasts when energy inside of them is activated and awakened.

In systems like Chinese Medicine and Yoga, there is mention of channels of energy that flow through the human body. All of us contain life force energy within. And that life force moves through a network of channels in our bodies. If we were to open a human body and take a look inside, we wouldn't be able to physically see these channels with our eyes. They're based in our subtle body and can really only be experienced by actually feeling them within ourselves.

Chinese Medicine looks at these channels as energy meridians and uses practices like acupuncture to directly work with these meridians. In Yoga, it is said that we each have seventy-two thousand of these energy channels in our bodies. When energy is flowing freely through them, we feel dynamic, energized, and at hone in our bodies. But when we have blocked energy inside, we might feel anxiety, fatigue, stagnation, or restlessness in our daily lives.

The breasts, like all the other parts of the body, carry their own energy channels. By using practices like self-massage, movement, stretching, dance, visualization, and meditation, the energy channels inside of the breasts can be cleared, which will, in turn, activate our breasts. Once your breasts are activated, you will start to feel a tingly, turned-on, and wild vibration circulating within your breasts and heart.

Since they're located near the heart, the breasts have a very direct connection to the frequency present within the heart.

*The energies of a woman's breasts and heart
are deeply interwoven. Together, they work to magnify
her power and potential.*

Science tells us that our heart carries the highest amount of electromagnetic frequency in the body. In fact, the heart is so powerful that its electromagnetic field is five thousand times greater than that of the brain's. The heart is an absolute powerhouse.

We can even use an electrocardiogram (ECG) to measure the energy of the heart as far as three feet from the body. That's how far the electromagnetic field of the heart is said to extend.[17]

Perhaps the heart's energy can even go out beyond three feet, and it's just that we lack the tools to measure at that distance.

---

17. Jessica I. Morales, "The Heart's Electromagnetic Field Is Your Superpower," *Psychology Today*, November 29, 2020, https://www.psychologytoday.com/us/blog/building-the-habit-hero/202011/the-hearts-electromagnetic-field-is-your-superpower.

Between the heart's out-of-this-world electromagnetic frequency and the breasts' energy channels, the result is an intoxicating mix of divine love, feminine-powered wisdom, and unrelenting compassion. In our day-to-day lives, we're too busy and not present enough in our bodies to notice the rich and vivid world that exists under our skin.

Our breasts show us who we are.

Once you unlock the frequencies in your heart and breasts, you will start to feel, at a deep cellular level, like the goddess you truly are.

Like the womb, our hearts can hold on to and carry stuck emotions and feelings we haven't yet processed and moved on from. Whether it's a breakup, losing a loved one, or being betrayed by another, every woman knows what it's like to experience pain in her heart. Words like *heartache* and *heartbreak* are literal ways of explaining the kind of pain we are sometimes forced to grapple with. When the heart experiences pain and struggle again and again and continues to hold on to these feelings, they can be held for years, even decades. As heartaches continue to pile up through a lifetime, without being processed, this can shut us down and desensitize us to all the connection and feelings in our breasts.

Some yogis believe this is one of the reasons why breast cancer is so prevalent. They believe that all the emotional burdens we carry in our hearts and breasts can impact our physical health and actually create disease and imbalance in the body.

When you start to work in partnership with your body, when you start to love every inch of your physical being, the conditions for greater wellness and balance are created. A vibrant kind of energy starts to emanate from your eyes and aura. You become fully acquainted with and infused by all the sensual, joyful, and radiant feminine energies that have always been inside of you.

Combining the energies of love from heart and breasts with the energies of creation and potential in the womb space makes for a force to be reckoned with.

Practice
Meditate on Your Breasts

To begin to activate your breasts, you must first sit in stillness and *feel into them.*

Be sure there are no distractions while you do this practice. Approaching these breast practices is sacred work, so be sure you're in a safe and quiet spot. Turn off your phone, close your door, and get comfortable.

If you're sitting, make sure to sit up with a straight spine. Start to take some womb breaths. Just allow your body to relax and let go.

With every exhale, feel your body relax even more deeply. Don't get frustrated if you're not able to focus. If thoughts appear, just gently bring yourself back to your breath and body.

Now, start to focus on both your left and your right breasts at the same time. And here's the important thing: you want to focus on both of them from the inside, and not the outside. Feel your breasts from within. Pick one point in each breast and stay settled there. Your focus should be nice and soft, and on both breasts at the same time.

Do this for ten minutes as you continue to breathe deeply.

As you practice this meditation, you might notice some sensation or vibration in your breasts, chest, or heart. If you do notice something, try to hone in on it. It means your energy channels are opening and that you're beginning to feel the spark of energy within you. Try to meditate on that spark as you continue to breathe.

You might experience emotion during this practice. If you feel like crying, and you're really not sure why, know this is perfectly normal. If you're just becoming acquainted with this part of yourself, you might connect with some unprocessed emotions that want to come up to the surface. If you feel safe to let go and cry, this will help move the emotions and clear your energy channels within.

If you don't feel anything or notice anything during or after this practice, don't get discouraged. Try it again the next day, and just show up, open to whatever rises to the surface.

Trust that you're exactly where you need to be right now, and that you've got this.

What You Focus on Expands

If you notice any sensations coming up during or after trying the breast meditation practice, try to continue breathing and focus on what is revealing itself to you. It might be a tingly kind of feeling. It might feel like a cool or warm sensation. It might be a vibration. As you work with your energy and your channels within, different kinds of feelings and sensations will start to make themselves known to you.

Since what we focus on expands, try to focus on what you're feeling once it comes. And keep on breathing and staying present. Allow this sensation, feeling, or vibration to bask in the light of your recognition and loving attention. Too often we skirt past the sensations and feelings in our bodies because we just don't have the time and the patience for them.

Part of developing a deeper connection to our wombs, breasts, and bodies is noticing what is happening inside of us each day. Sometimes that is as simple as having daily check-ins with ourselves—stopping what we're doing to just breathe and scan our bodies to see what is present there.

Owning your power means taking everything off autopilot. It means devoting yourself to each and every sensation, fluttering, vibration, and whisper within.

Once you start becoming more mindful of what's happening in your body, you will start to notice things there that you never knew existed. You might start to realize that your ability to feel pleasure is much higher than it was, or that you've got this unshakable sense of self-love that's been part of you this entire time. It might unearth this inner confidence that starts as a tiny spark within, but then expands outward, its effects spreading into every single thing you do.

All the electromagnetic energy in the heart is like a gift. We just have to know how to receive it. Having such high frequency in the heart space means there's a door of potential, a chance to start developing our awareness of the energy that is present and available there.

BREAST MASSAGE

There's nothing on this earth I love doing more than breast massage. I can't think of a more healing, restorative, and pleasurable practice for women.

If you're ever having a bad day, ask yourself: Did I give myself a breast massage this morning? Chances are, you didn't!

When you start your day with breast massage, nothing can go wrong. It's like you're bulletproof. It's like you have this mega-powerful force field around you that zaps all the negativity away. Your breasts are superpowers, and when they're activated, all your magnetic, confident, joyful, and radiant energies will come up to the surface.

The only message we've ever been given when it comes to touching our breasts has to do with checking them for lumps, in case the threat of breast cancer is present.

How can women truly create more balance, wellness, and health within the body if they're only told to touch their breasts to make sure they don't have cancer? How much more disempowering does it have to get before all women start to break away from the old stories and come back to their wild, natural, primal, and glorious selves?

Checking for lumps in your breasts is a wise thing to do, but it can't be everything. It won't sustain and rejuvenate your heart and spirit in the ways you deeply deserve.

Our breasts need nourishment, love, and care.

As the vessels that hold, in part, the high frequencies of our unconditional love, immunity, and compassion, our breasts are desperately craving our touch and attention. Breast massage is the path to really caring for body, mind, and spirit. It's the path to reclaiming part of your beautiful feminine body and opening up to the ocean of potential that flows within you.

Breast massage carries all sorts of healing, therapeutic benefits as well. It's a great way of stimulating the lymphatic system and helping our bodies push out toxins, reduce inflammation, and boost immunity. Breast massage also stimulates blood circulation and can help relieve pain and stress. It even works wonders for firming and toning the breasts.

The beauty of breast massage is that it doesn't have to be some whole big production that requires candles, incense, 52-hertz music playing in the background, and seven different exotic oils. You don't even have to take your shirt off if you don't want to, or if you don't have time to.

I do the majority of my breast massages with my shirt on and no oil, which is what I've found works best for me. Also, between having work and family to devote my attention to, I need self-care practices that are convenient and quick while packing a tremendous punch in the process.

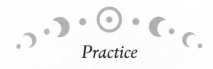

Practice

Breast Massage #1
(Low Maintenance)

Do this practice first thing in the morning, if you can. You only have to devote a few minutes to this low-maintenance practice. You can always go longer, if you like. Since women are often so busy juggling different responsibilities, I like to share effective practices that can make an impact without eating up too much time.

For the first time you practice this, however, I suggest you set aside at least ten to twenty minutes. If you aren't accustomed to breast massage, it's a good idea to get in a solid first session where you really start to connect with your breasts. After you get a substantial first session in, you can go for quick two- to three-minute sessions in the future. It's a great thing to do each morning before you leave for work or start your day.

For this practice, you don't need any oil, and you don't need to remove your top.

Before you start, one thing to keep in mind: when doing this particular breast massage routine, be sure to always stroke away from the body and not toward the centerline of your body. The channels of energy located in the chest and heart region extend outward. When you massage in an outward direction, you're working in alignment with those channels, which will increase your odds of clearing stuck energies.

From a seated position, take a few deep womb breaths through the nose to connect to your body.

Cup your left breast in your left hand, and cup your right breast in your right hand. Give your breasts a nice, gentle shake, up and down, as you continue to cup them. Be sure to keep breathing deeply as you do this. Make sure all your muscles are relaxed.

Bring the fingers of both hands to the center of your chest, just underneath your collarbone. Start to massage by making outward circles. As you massage, slowly start to move your left and right hands farther apart from each other, toward your underarms. You can stop once you reach the underarm area.

Now, start in the middle again, except this time, move down half an inch so you can cover a new area. Massage from the center all the way across your chest. Continue doing this until you make it all the way to your breasts.

Once you get to your breasts, massage them at the same time, with left hand massaging left breast, and right hand massaging right breast. Make big circles that move in the outer direction, instead of circles that go in toward the centerline of the body. As you do this, be sure to keep your palms against your breasts. You want to be completely relaxed.

Continue the massage, using your natural instinct to determine how to touch your chest and breasts.

This is deep, sacred work. When you do this, you're clearing energy channels, which may be holding a lot of stuck emotions and feelings. If you cry during the massage, it just means your energy channels are releasing what needs to be released. Take it slow, be gentle with yourself, and don't forget to breathe!

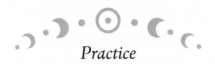

Practice

Breast Massage #2
(Not So Low Maintenance)

This second breast massage is for those days when you have more time and want to go all out. It involves setting up the perfect environment, removing your top and bra, and whipping out some massage oil. I probably make time to do this kind of breast massage once every few months. But if it resonates with you, and you don't mind all the extra effort, *go for it*. Do this as often as you like. When breast massage is involved, the phrase "too much of a good thing" simply does not apply. And you can quote me on that.

Plan to set aside about half an hour for this practice. Go someplace where you won't be disturbed. Make sure it's quiet and comfortable. Set the right environment for your breast massage. Whatever makes you feel most relaxed. You can light a candle or some incense, play some relaxing music in the background, turn on an aromatherapy diffuser, or even sage the room before you begin.

Find a massage oil that is safe to work with on the skin. If you don't have a massage oil, good old olive oil works just fine. In the past, I've worked with olive oil, sesame oil, and grapeseed oil for my massages. All of them felt heavenly, and they have their own unique element they bring to the massage.

Set up a towel underneath you in case the oil spills onto your floor, bed, chair, or any other surface you might be resting on.

Remove any top and bra so your breasts are free.

You can either lie down or sit up for this. Again, do what feels amazing and right for you and your body.

Place both of your hands (without the oil) over your heart, and just stay here for a couple of minutes. Start to take womb breaths, breathing down deep into the womb, as you start to connect to the heart and feel what's transpiring within it.

Now, when you feel connected, take your oil and put some on your hands. Start to massage your chest and breast area with the palms of both your left and right hands, making big circles that extend in a direction away from the centerline of your body.

Start to use your fingers to massage outward circles across your chest; go from just below the collarbone and work your way to the breasts.

After massaging outward circles on your breasts, mix it up a bit by squeezing both breasts at the same time, using a pressure that feels pleasurable to you. Take left breast in left hand, and right breast in right hand, and squeeze.

Use your instincts in massaging your chest and breasts. Find the rhythm and techniques that work for you and your body.

Toward the end of the massage, take your right hand across and use the palm to massage the left side of the chest. Then ease that motion all the way out toward the arm, massaging down the arm to the wrist. Repeat this on the other side.

As you do this breast massage, take your time. No rushing. Luxuriate in each moment, allowing the medicine of the breast massage to heal, restore, and nourish you. Let that vibrant, unapologetic goddess inside of you come to life.

The more you massage your breasts, the more alive, balanced, and loving you'll feel. You'll start to feel as if your heart and breasts are infused with sunshine. This kind of aliveness, this kind of plea-sure—it's something you deserve to know and feel on a daily basis.

When I tell women that a consistent breast massage practice is one of the most life-changing things they can ever do for themselves, they will sometimes laugh. They think I'm joking, but I would never joke about breast massage—it's serious business! Give yourself a breast massage every day for five minutes a day, thirty days straight; and then you'll know what I'm talking about.

CREATING A BRIDGE BETWEEN BREASTS AND WOMB

Paying attention to our feminine parts is beyond empowering. Many of us haven't been taught to acknowledge ourselves in this way. This has caused a great deal of guilt, shame, disconnect, and confusion to build up in our bod-ies, distancing us from knowing and trusting in our authentic selves.

Diving deep into the power of womb, breasts, and body deepens connec-tion to the self. It brings you to a place of realization, so that you can intimately interact with all the sacredness, all the magic, all the divinity you hold within. In this lifetime, you deserve to be aligned to this natural state.

Deepen your connection to the body, and the nature of your authentic self will become known to you.

Since the heart is the space of love and the place in the body where elec-tromagnetic energy is highest, this is the starting point. This is the spark that boldly dares to make itself known, before it dances itself into a beautiful, brilliant fire within.

Once we can feel the explosive energy of the heart and breasts, we might start to notice more subtle kinds of energy running through our bodies. This high frequency of the heart can then be channeled into the womb, enhanc-ing the uterus with the energies of love and compassion. Creating a bridge between these two power sources is a key part of owning the potential that is abundantly inherent in your inner feminine landscape.

Practice

Connecting Breasts and Womb

As always, find a quiet and comfortable place to sit.

Place your left hand on your heart and your right hand on the womb.

Sit here for a few moments and take a few deep womb breaths. Pay attention to what's happening within you. Situate your attention into the center of your heart and just breathe.

Now, focus on the insides of both your left and right breasts. Pick a point within each one, and stay settled there. Once you find that point, try your best not to stray from it. Continue your womb breaths as you stay settled here, focusing on the insides of both left and right breasts.

After a few minutes, or when you're sure you feel a strong connection with your breasts and heart, you can let go of this part of the practice.

Next, take a deep inhale while imagining you're guiding your breath from the heart all the way down into the womb.

On your exhale, you will do the opposite. As you exhale deeply out the nose, you're envisioning that the breath is moving from the womb and to the heart. Try to keep this going for five to ten minutes.

What you're doing here is creating a circuit of energy. The breath is moving, unbroken, in a circular type of fashion between heart and womb. Continue circulating your energy between the two. And be sure to breathe slowly and deeply as you do this. Take your time and allow yourself to melt into the moment.

NOW WHAT?

Once you've opened the door to your heart and breasts in this way, there's no limit to what you can do. Your body, mind, and spirit are propelled to this whole other level where balance, inner peace, and joy are readily available to you. As you continue to deepen your connection to your breasts, you'll naturally become present to all the vibrancy inside your body.

Here are some other ways to liberate and activate the energy of your breasts:

- Jump on a trampoline if you have access to one! As you do, make a conscious effort to focus on your breasts. Jumping on a trampoline is a great way to get the breasts in motion, allowing them to clear and release stagnant energy.
- Do a stretch to open and activate the chest area. Stand in an open doorway, holding the frame with your right hand. Twist and look toward the left. You should feel the stretch on the right side of your chest. Stay like this for thirty seconds, and then do the other side.
- Make arm circles to activate heart, breasts, and chest. Make large arm circles forward fifteen times, and then backward fifteen times.
- Speak a positive affirmation to your breasts at the start of your day. Place your hands over your breasts, take a deep breath, and say, "My breasts are beautiful."
- Before you get in the shower, take time to look at your bare breasts in the mirror. Do some womb breathing as you look at your breasts. Let any feelings come up to the surface. If you notice that you feel uncomfortable, know this is normal. Many of us aren't used to showing our breasts any kind of attention, and when we do, we often tend to focus on the things we don't like. This time, though, you're flipping the script. You're choosing to acknowledge your breasts, along with all the beauty and power they hold.
- Remember to try to do a quick breast massage every day, if you can!
- Meditate on the breasts at least once a week or every other week.
- Eat nutritious foods to keep your breasts healthy. Whole grains, vegetables, fruits, nuts, and foods rich in omega-3s (like chia seeds and walnuts) are all great options.

Journal Prompts
Knowing Your Breasts

Finally, write about your breasts in your Womb Journal. Your breasts play a significant role in this journey toward womb wellness. So, carve out some time to journal about your current relationship to your breasts. Write the answers to questions like:

- How do I interact with my breasts throughout the day, if I do at all?
- What do I think about my breasts?
- What has shaped my attitude toward my breasts?
- How can I show my breasts more love, care, and attention?

When you journal about anything, in general, practice trying to feel the words pour from your heart and breasts, down your arms and hands, and onto the paper. This practice will help you more deeply bring out your thoughts, feelings, and revelations. It will bring you to a space of interlocking your inner and outer worlds and allow you to truly write from the heart, to let what's inside of you come out onto the page. This is also a very cleansing and nourishing practice for the breasts.

When you can start feeling that divine connection with your heart and breasts, and you can actually bring that connection directly into what you're doing, speaking, writing, or creating, you will be engaging in one of the purest forms of expression imaginable.

Start writing from your heart, literally, and you will notice the difference in how your words and sentence structures fill the pages.

Having a picture of what has transpired for you will really help you heal and evolve. Be sure to write in your journal after doing things like breast massage, breast meditation, and other practices. This will help you track everything and see how far you've come.

When I started working with my breasts and womb in a more intentional way, all kinds of sensations and transformations occurred within me. And it all happened so fast. In the moment, things might feel really potent and explosive. But then, over time, we may forget all the details of our experiences. Capturing them in your journal is a key way to document your journey and to help propel you to the next steps.

CHAPTER 7 TAKEAWAYS

- Our breasts are for so much more than breastfeeding or attracting and pleasing others. Women must start practicing self-care for the breasts in order to fully know their power.
- The heart contains the highest amount of electromagnetic frequency in the body. As the breasts are an extension of the heart, they carry this energy, too.
- Breast massage, meditation, and other practices are essential for aligning to and amplifying our feminine energy.
- A quick morning breast massage (without oil or the need to remove your shirt) is an empowering way to start the day.
- Breast energy must be bridged to womb energy in order for women to experience a depth of love, pleasure, and fulfillment.
- Plugging into heart energy and letting it flow out onto the paper during journaling is a must.

Chapter 8

VAGINA

"The ancient Taoists regarded the feminine genitalia with respect and admired her natural beauty. They studied her landscape as an art and science."
—Minke de Vos[18]

When I was younger, I had always thought the vagina was the outer part—the place where the lips and the vulva were, the place you could easily touch and see with your own eyes.

But as I got older, I realized that what I had always thought of and referred to as my vagina wasn't really my vagina at all. I learned my vagina was actually on the inside, an inner canal that connected to the bottom of the uterus and the top of the cervix.

This just about blew my mind.

Isn't it strange how such an intimate part of ourselves can sometimes be so unknown and foreign to us? Our vaginas play such a necessary role in our bodies, and yet, just as we do with our wombs, we don't really think about them all that much. Though they are part of our bodies, we exist at a remove from them, only focusing on them during times of menstruation, childbirth, and sex.

This could be due, in part, to the fact that we're simply not taught, at a young age, about the true sacredness and power inherent in our feminine

18. Vos, *Tao Tantric Arts for Women*, 177.

bodies. Some of us have experienced sexual traumas, emotional pain, or physical issues that have kept us from connecting with this part of ourselves.

Whatever the case may be, it's never too late to start knowing your vagina in a deeper, more intimate way.

Why Would I Want To?

Thousands of years ago, there were ancient cultures that understood the wisdom and sacredness inherent in the vagina and womb. In places throughout India, for example, they created statues, erected temples, and held ceremonies to honor and revere the vagina and the part it plays in bringing life into the world.

But this wisdom has been lost over time.

Many years later, women find themselves disconnected or numb to the inner callings of their vaginas and wombs. Our fast-paced world has forgotten the mysteries of the feminine. We've fallen out of alignment with the cycles and rhythms of the earth, moon, and nature.

The good news is that this wisdom, although buried, is still present there. Our vaginas hold this wisdom, just as our wombs do. As an integral part of our feminine bodies, our vaginas are passageways, places through which menstrual blood and babies move. The role that our vaginas play in bringing our precious creations into the world is immense.

Your vagina is the bridge between your inner and outer worlds; it's what connects your womb to the environment around you.

As a "middlewoman," your vagina holds the balance between the seen and unseen, between what is imagined and what is physically manifested.

Your vagina is also the place that welcomes in a lover. And any lover that is taken into the vagina leaves their energy within its walls. This is why, as women, we must be mindful of whom we let inside of us. Their emotions come into us when they "cum" into us. And even when there is no ejaculation, the energies from their genitals still linger inside of us.

This is why it can sometimes be tough to move on and cut ties with a lover you want to get out of your life. It's also why, even after you've removed a toxic lover from your life, you still feel weighted down by their energies. This person could be all the way on the other side of the world, yet their energy can still zap you into feeling off-balance, sad, lonely, emotional, and pining for your old lover.

Just as the womb can hold on to emotions and energies, so can the vagina. As they operate and work together, one can impact the other in profound ways. The healing you do in your vagina affects the womb—and the healing you do in your womb affects the vagina.

Becoming more conscious of your vagina allows your feminine nature to be liberated. It gives you a deep connection to the goddess within—the one who is connected to her sensuality, her purpose, and her confidence. The one who celebrates herself and her body each and every single day. The one who lights up every room she walks into, because all the vitality, all the love inside of her, is like an intoxicating avalanche of expression.

Since your vagina is what brings womb and outer world into relationship, keeping her clear and vibrant is a must. She is the conduit, the place through which the wild river of your soul and womb flow out to touch the world. Otherwise, your feminine expression is locked and sealed tightly in the womb. This might feel good to hold in your body for a little while. You will feel the electricity of the womb within you, and it will be a beautiful revelation of the power you hold. But without the vagina, it goes nowhere. It sits stagnant in the womb. And just as anything that sits stagnant, it can become toxic over time.

Your vagina provides the outlet, the opening, the way forward. It brings the expression of the womb out into the world. It blesses the world with your love, your intention, and your power. It gives life to every gesture blossoming within the wild terrain of your womb space.

What you want to create, birth, or manifest—all of that is nurtured in the womb. Once all of that is ready to be brought out into the world, the vagina is the energetic space, the part of you that transports your inner fire onto the outer plane.

Our bodies are wonders to behold. Every part of ourselves plays a role in keeping us activated, healthy, balanced, and alive. Although this is happening automatically within us every day, we must not take a bit of it for granted. We must make the time to honor and cherish each and every part of ourselves.

Our vaginas aren't appreciated nearly enough for the work they do. We might pay attention to them when we're menstruating, or when we're deep in concentration as we push a baby out, or when we're taking a lover inside of us. But if we're only noticing our vaginas during these times, we're doing ourselves a disservice. We're not giving ourselves the opportunity to become conscious and aware of what's happening inside of the vagina, and what emotions or energies we might need to clear and release.

If you feel you haven't ever been really connected to your vagina, take some time to understand why that is. All of us have our own stories, our own reasons, for disconnecting from our bodies or shutting down certain parts of ourselves. Understand what your stories are, and how they've impacted your relationship with your vagina.

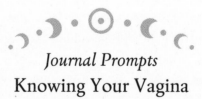

Journal Prompts
Knowing Your Vagina

Start asking yourself questions, and write down whatever answers come up. Drink some water before you write, and allow the words to flow from your heart, without trying to control them. Let your responses be raw and full of truth.

- What is my current relationship with my vagina?
- What kinds of experiences have happened in my life to impact my relationship with my vagina?

- How do I currently feel about my vagina?
- And how do I want to feel about my vagina moving forward?

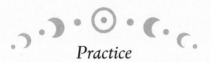

Practice
First Connection with the Vagina

To build a relationship with your vagina, you have to first be able to imagine and feel it within you. Once you connect with it in this way, you can start to understand where it's located internally and actually notice it in your body as it does its important work.

Try this practice…

Find a comfortable place to lie down.

Start to take some deep womb breaths, and just allow your body to soften and relax.

Feel everything in your pelvis melting and relaxing. Let your womb be open and soft.

Now focus your attention into the entrance of your vagina. Settle here and just allow yourself to feel what's happening in this space. Take deep womb breaths and let yourself melt and relax right here at the vaginal entrance.

After a few minutes, allow your mind to move from the entrance and into the vagina. Let yourself go in about an inch. Stop here and notice what you feel. Notice how different being inside of the vagina might feel from being right at the entrance. Continue to do your womb breaths here and just allow yourself to drop all your energy into this space.

Now, try to go up even deeper into the vagina, toward the womb. The average length of the vagina is about three to four inches. (This can actually expand to five to six inches when you're aroused.) Go in another couple of inches, until you are at the bottom of the cervix, which is the lower portion of the uterus. Remember, you're just using your imagination for this practice, and not physically touching yourself.

Now rest here, and continue to take womb breaths. Feel into this deep part of the vagina and breathe. Notice any other differences in sensation you might feel in this area.

When you're finished, be sure to journal about how this practice made you feel. In some cases, you might have noticed differences between the various parts of the vagina. Maybe you didn't notice anything, or maybe it was hard for you to concentrate. Trust that your unique experience was perfect for you and where you are in your journey.

Try to repeat this weekly to give yourself the time and space to get to know and understand your vagina more intimately.

FEELING YOUR VAGINA

A deeper way of knowing the vagina is through touch.

The thought of this might ignite a little fear or uncertainty within, which is perfectly understandable.

Women aren't used to exploring themselves and touching their intimate parts. We often think of these parts only under the banner of sexual encounters, which is a very limited way of knowing what we and our bodies are capable of.

To really understand and explore your vagina, you must approach it with an open heart and mind and a willingness to put aside any preconceived notions of what touching your vagina might mean.

Blessing your vagina with touch is a sign of love, respect, and appreciation for your own body and self. It's a way of owning your power, sensuality, vitality, and birthright as a woman.

Touching your vagina may seem strange and unnatural at first, if it isn't something you're accustomed to doing. But if you make time to practice this, your vagina and body will start getting used to it. And not only that, but you'll start to feel more energy, vitality, and clarity radiating through your vagina.

Conjure up the image of a woman touching her vagina in your mind. *What do you see?*

Most likely you're imagining the woman is giving herself sexual pleasure. This is because something as simple as touching our vaginas hasn't been normalized or accepted as a way of understanding and knowing ourselves. It is only thought of in a sexual context.

Of course, there's nothing wrong about a woman pleasuring herself and touching her vagina! In fact, many of us women could use a little more self-pleasuring in our lives. But touching our vaginas is more than just sexual gratification—at least in the context of this chapter. When you give your vagina your touch, you are giving yourself a wider, more in-depth understanding of who you are as a woman. You're also opening yourself up to who you might become as you lock into the core parts of yourself, the parts of yourself that house all your precious power.

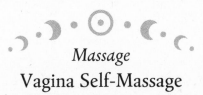

Massage
Vagina Self-Massage

Using touch, or self-massage, to connect to the vagina is an empowering practice. It might feel kind of weird at first, but as your body softens and relaxes, you'll be able to get into it more and notice the sensations that arise.

Massaging the vagina is an act of self-love. It has the potential to free up the space of any stuck emotions or toxic forms of energy you might be holding on to from past lovers or negative sexual encounters.

If the thought of massaging your vagina makes you feel uncomfortable, don't force yourself into it. Put it off for a while, until you feel you're mentally or emotionally ready. You can even just, for the first time, focus on the opening of the vagina if you're not fully ready to go inside. Working with our vaginal opening also offers a great deal of healing and energetic release.

To start, set up your environment in such a way that makes you feel honored. Clean up your space and light some candles or incense. Play some relaxing music, if you like.

Take off any bottoms and underwear. You can place a blanket over your lower half if you feel cold, or if you just want something to cover you.

When you're ready, follow these steps for the massage ...

Lie down on your back and make sure you're comfortable. Remember to do your womb breaths to relax your body and mind.

Now, take your index finger and place it gently over the entrance of your vagina. Continue the womb breaths here as you focus on the entrance. Notice the way the entrance feels with your finger against it.

Next, take a deep breath. As you do so, start to slowly insert your finger into your vagina. Stop when you've reached about an inch. And now just take a moment to notice what you feel. At this point, you aren't doing any kind of massaging yet. You're just noticing what it feels like to have your own finger an inch into your vagina. As you notice, don't forget to breathe.

Start to very slowly and softly massage the inside of the vagina, making circular motions with your finger. Feel all around your vagina as you do so.

The important thing is to keep breathing as you do this. Take a moment to notice your entire body. If you're holding any tension anywhere in your body, it will have an impact on this practice, and could cut off the potential for more sensation and healing. So, try to consciously relax the other parts of your body. As you relax the other parts of your body, your vagina will follow suit.

As you continue to massage, breathe and just let yourself be aware and conscious of what you're feeling moment-to-moment. You might notice some tender spots. These are the places where your vagina is storing and holding on to stuck energies and emotions. Be extra conscious and slow down when navigating these areas.

From here, you can stop the self-massage practice, especially if it's your first time doing it.

Next time, you can always challenge yourself to go a little deeper. I'm a big believer of going slow, and not suddenly overwhelming the body with new practices and sensations. However, if you feel ready to move on, go ahead and press your finger a half inch or an inch deeper into your vagina. Continue the same massaging movement as you breathe, and stay present to all you're feeling.

After the massage, take some time to lie down in silence and notice what your vagina, womb, and body feel like. Take some time to journal about it, so that you can go back later in your journey to remember what self-massaging your vagina felt like in the beginning. That way, you can compare your feelings as you get further along in your journey.

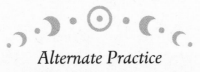

Alternate Practice
Self-Massage for Your Pelvis

Massaging the inside of the vagina might not be possible for some women. If you're a trans woman, or you've experienced sexual trauma in the vagina, or you have a medical condition, like vaginismus or vulvar vestibulitis, you might want to try an alternative massage that is just as healing and transformative.

This pelvic massage involves touch on the outside of the pelvis. Your pelvis is located below the belly button, between your abdomen and thighs; it contains the reproductive organs and bladder. This part of ourselves is often neglected, though it works so hard every day to provide our digestive and reproductive systems support and balance. Offering touch to this area is incredibly healing. Be sure to find a pressure that works for you and your body. This self-massage can even be done with a feather-light touch, while still delivering deep healing and relaxation.

Lie down on your back and make sure you're comfortable. Remember to do your womb breaths to relax your body and mind.

Place your hands and fingers in a downward-facing triangle, right below your belly button. The tips of your thumbs should be touching and positioned directly under the belly button. The tips of your index fingers should be touching as well. This should form a downward-facing triangle right over your pelvis.

Breathe here and feel the power of your pelvis radiating beneath your hands and fingers.

Now, keeping your fingers in the triangular formation, start to lightly massage the pelvis.

Breathe deep into your womb as you massage, and allow yourself to be completely immersed in whatever feelings or sensations come up.

Whenever you're ready to move on, you can release the triangle formation and do some freestyle massage over the pelvis. You might want to spend a little extra time on areas that feel good or are a little tender. Remember to use whatever pressure feels good and safe for you so you can relax fully and explore this part of yourself.

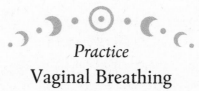

Practice

Vaginal Breathing

This vaginal breathing practice is a great way to calm your nervous system down and bring ease into your body. Engaging in vaginal breathing can also make you more in tune with what's happening inside of your vagina, while also helping relieve any tension or stuck feelings you might be having there.

Sit up with a straight spine and get those womb breaths going.

Give yourself a minute to let your body relax and your mind wind down.

When you're ready, imagine your vagina is actually inhaling the next breath. So, as you inhale, imagine your vagina is pulling that breath in through its canal and up into the womb.

At the end of the inhale, hold your breath in your womb as you concentrate on the center of the uterus.

When you exhale, imagine you are breathing that breath down from the womb, down the vaginal canal, and out of the body.

With the exhale, give yourself the opportunity of feeling your womb, vagina, and all reproductive organs completely soften and release anything they may be holding on to.

Do this breath as many times as you like.

Yoni Eggs

Some women swear by using yoni eggs to clear and cleanse the energies in the vagina. Yoni eggs are crystals you insert into the vagina to help restore and shift energy. Some of the eggs are drilled with a hole inside of them, and so they have a string at the end, which you can use to tug the egg out when you're finished. Others have no holes or strings attached, so you would have to simply push the egg out of the vagina when you're done.

Once the egg is inside of your vagina, you can meditate, do Kegels, visualize, or do some deep breathing exercises. Depending upon what kind of crystal you choose, that crystal will infuse the vagina with its energy and bring its healing attributes into your sacred space.

There are many sellers offering yoni eggs, but not all of them are of high quality. If you're interested in purchasing a yoni egg, be sure to buy it from a seller who uses high-quality crystals in their products. Otherwise your yoni egg will carry very low vibrations and won't end up having much of an effect.

If you do decide to use yoni eggs, it's important to keep them clean. Be sure to wash them thoroughly before and after you use them so bacteria cannot form and cause any infections in the body.

Vaginal Steaming

Vaginal steaming, or yoni steaming, has been all the rage over these last several years. Many new spas are adding it to their menus as women are looking for treatments that go deeper to heal the womb and vagina. Involving the use of herbs to steam the vagina and womb, vaginal steaming offers countless benefits. See chapter 9 to learn more in-depth information about how to do a steam on your own.

Vaginal Love

At the end of the day, your vagina needs your love. It's a vibrant part of who you are, and it is brimming with all kinds of endless potential. It's a wise, all-knowing force that is in direct relationship with your womb and the outer world. All day it flows with vital information. Make time during your days to stop whatever it is you're doing and just feel into your vagina and your pelvis. Give your vagina your love, your attention, and your focus. Show it that you value all the many things it does to sustain and nurture you.

Love for this part of yourself isn't something that has to be far away. It's something you can feel *now*. It's something you can realize in this moment.

And in turn, your vagina will heal and thrive. Respect, celebrate, and appreciate your vagina, and you will feel the power and confidence within you magnify tenfold.

Chapter 8 Takeaways

- Your vagina is what connects your womb to the outer world. It's an essential kind of bridge that brings your creations and your essence into full expression.
- Honoring and caring for the vagina has an impact on the womb, and honoring and caring for the womb affects the vagina as well. Heal one, and you heal the other.
- Since our vaginas are so often ignored outside the context of sex, menstruation, and childbirth, we must start to form a relationship

with them. One of the best ways to start is by journaling. Using meditation and self-massage are other beneficial ways of healing and nurturing the vagina.

- You can take matters into your own hands and demonstrate love for your vagina *today*. By celebrating your vagina, you celebrate yourself and amplify your power.

Chapter 9

VAGINAL STEAMING

"Yoni Steaming assists us in doing all that is within our power to restore our lives and our wombs to a state of health and balance."
  —Iya Olosunde Ajala[19]

NOTE: If you don't have a yoni to steam, you can still take part in this practice by using the pelvis as your focus. Just as the womb is an energetic space all of us contain within, the yoni is the same. Even without a yoni, you can follow all the steps in doing a yoni steam and still reap the healing benefits.

The first time I ever tried a yoni steam, I was like, *Where have you been all my life?*

I'd never felt such relaxation *down there*.

Imagine that every single muscle, nerve, and cell in your womb and vagina felt as if they were all breathing out a sigh of tremendous relief, as if years of stagnant energy and emotion were all melting away in one deep release, and that'll give you some approximation of how I felt during that first yoni steam. In all the yoni steaming I've done after that, I've been astounded by how that feeling has continued.

Yoni steaming—also known as vaginal steaming, V-steaming, or pelvic steaming—is a soothing, rejuvenating practice that involves using hot water and herbs to steam the vagina. *Yoni* is an ancient Sanskrit word that

---

19. Iya Olosunde Ajala, *Yoni Steam* (Self-published, 2015), 13.

can actually refer to three different parts of our feminine bodies. Depending on who you're talking to, *yoni* means "vagina," "vulva," or "womb." When I use the word *yoni*, I often think of it as being the vagina. Throughout the centuries, yoni steaming has been practiced by different cultures in places like Africa, Asia, and South America. Indigenous women have been steaming their yonis since way back, long before Gwyneth Paltrow made headlines with her yoni steam back in 2015.[20]

Although this has been a practice that has been embraced since ancient times, many people jumped all over Paltrow after learning about her yoni steams, saying that steaming wasn't proven to be of much benefit at all. Many hinged their theory on the idea that the vagina self-cleans, so women don't need a steam for cleaning.

However, a yoni steam isn't so much about cleaning the vagina and womb. It's more about taking the benefits of the herbs and, through the water vapor, delivering those benefits to the feminine parts of our bodies.

Steaming the yoni isn't just some passing fad. It's a restorative practice that not only promotes deep relaxation, but also has the ability to bring about major transformation and healing.

WHY EVEN BOTHER?

Over five thousand years ago, the Sumerians, who lived in ancient Mesopotamia, used clay tablets to record their findings on two hundred fifty plants and twelve herbal recipes. This is the oldest written record that exists on herbs. In the ancient Egyptians' Papyrus, during about 1500 BCE, they also included references to eight hundred fifty herbal remedies, which include herbs we know today, like aloe, cedar, and cumin.

In India, a healing medicine practice known as Ayurveda began several thousand years ago. Ancient texts on Ayurveda have also been discovered,

---

20. US Weekly Staff, "Gwyneth Paltrow Gets Vaginal Steam at Spa, Preaches its Virtues on Goop," *US Weekly,* January 29, 2015, https://www.usmagazine.com/stylish/news /gwyneth-paltrow-gets-vagina-steam-at-spa-preaches-its-virtues-on-goop-2015291/.

detailing hundreds of herbs and their uses. Chinese Medicine is another practice that has relied on and documented the power of herbs over the centuries.

Herbs have been used to treat illnesses, heal pain, balance the body, cure insomnia, and alleviate stress. Herbalism today is widely practiced and accepted, as more and more people in the world have experienced profound benefits from working with herbs.

Yoni steaming is just another way to enjoy the benefits of herbal magic. But why even do all this at all? Why even bother blasting herbs and steam into your yoni?

For starters, yoni steaming can:

- Bring healing to the uterus and vagina
- Promote fertility
- Relax the body
- Regulate menstruation
- Detoxify the womb
- Enhance sensuality and pleasure
- Balance emotions
- Balance hormones
- Cleanse the body of toxins
- Boost immunity
- Relieve stress

If you struggle with ovarian cysts, uterine fibroids, endometriosis, uterine prolapse, or postpartum issues like vaginal tearing or C-section scarring, yoni steaming might also be helpful for your healing process by bringing comfort and nourishment. Not to mention, it feels absolutely incredible while you're receiving it. For that reason alone, it's a worthwhile practice to consider. I also want to add that there haven't been any scientific studies done on yoni steaming, and that it probably isn't going to magically cure you of any serious medical conditions. But it's definitely a good self-care tool to use whenever you need it.

Yoni steaming is like a self-care spa for your womb and yoni. The steam delivers the herbs straight to your feminine parts so that your womb, vulva, and yoni can get the direct benefit from the herbal concoction of your choice. It's a deep cleanse of all the leftover residue from toxic situations, relationships, emotions, and experiences that have been energetically held inside of you.

You can absolutely access the power of herbs by sipping on some raspberry leaf tea, mixing some fresh rosemary into your stir-fry, or massaging your feet with some lavender oil. But in terms of healing and nurturing your womb, none of those come close to offering the benefits that steaming the yoni directly with herbs can provide.

When women steam their yonis, they fall into alignment with parts of themselves that are often neglected.

As women, we can sometimes pour lots of attention into doing things that will affect our outward appearance, like getting our nails done, doing our hair, or working out. There's nothing wrong with wanting to look good on the outside, *but what about the inside?* What about our wombs and vaginas, which go through so much during our lifetimes?

When a woman steams, she's telling her womb and vagina that they matter. She's showering love, attention, and energy toward her body, despite the cultural messages that her womb and vagina don't need this kind of nurturing, that they aren't worth the time or the bother.

But our wombs and our vaginas *are* worth it. *You are worth it.* You are sacred, your body is sacred, your womb is sacred, your vulva is sacred, and your vagina is sacred. And what is sacred deserves your unwavering love and attention. This is something you don't ever need to justify or apologize for.

PREPARING TO DO A YONI STEAM

Many spas are starting to offer yoni steams on the menu, so if you want to try one, you can try to look for a place near you. However, if there aren't any places near you, or you simply would like to try to do it yourself, yoni steaming can be done in the comfort of your own home. I do all my yoni steams at home and enjoy the ability to be flexible and comfortable in my own environment. I can light candles, play music I like, journal, and even speak affirmations as I'm doing my yoni steam.

If you want to learn how to do a yoni steam at home, it's very simple. The first thing you have to do is determine what you'll use for steaming. In the beginning of my yoni steaming journey, I went completely old school. I grabbed a huge pot and put it on the stove on high heat. Once it started to boil, I turned it off and just let it sit for several minutes. I didn't want to burn myself, so I had to make sure the water wasn't too hot. After that, I threw a handful of herbs in from my garden and just squatted over the pot, with a towel in my lap.

That's what I did in the beginning, because I just wanted to dive in and do it right away. I didn't want to waste time or money looking for the right supplies. My first experience was a bit haphazard, albeit enjoyable during the end result. But for anyone doing this for the first time, you'll have a deeper experience by being a bit more thoughtful about your setup than I was! Plus, looking back, what I did wasn't exactly the safest way to go about it. What if my leg muscles suddenly had gotten tired and I'd fallen into the pot?! It never happened, but it could've. So, protect your yoni, and don't do what I did.

SUGGESTED ITEMS FOR YONI STEAMING

Following is a list of recommended items you can prepare to do your yoni steam with, along with some suggested herbs to use. If you can't get access to all these items, there are alternatives for each.

Hot plate: This can be a basic plate you plug in with settings for temperature. If you don't have a hot plate, you can always just use your stove to heat up the water.

Pot: Any pot will do. Ideally, you should have a dedicated pot for yoni steaming. The optics might be a little wonky if you use the same pot for cooking your spaghetti and caring for your vagina.

Seat for yoni steaming (preferably a box-shaped seat with a hole in the middle): You can find yoni steam seats like this online, but it can cost about two hundred or three hundred dollars. Instead of this seat, you can also use a lawn chair that has openings underneath.

Gown: During your yoni steam, you'll need to have something to cover yourself while trapping all the heat. Gowns are comfortable, and if you don't have one, you can grab an inexpensive one online. You can also use a towel and drape it over the lower part of your body.

Herbs: Pick a few herbs based on what you want to get out of your yoni steaming session. You will need to add about a cup of herbs to your steam. Whether it's something like relaxation, fertility, or healing, there are countless herbs for many different needs. You can buy them separately and mix them together. Or there are some places online that sell herbal blends specifically made for yoni steams. If you grow herbs like I do, you can pick them from your own yard and toss them into your pot.

About a gallon of water.

SUGGESTED HERBS FOR YONI STEAMING

This is a list of some of my favorite herbs to use for steaming. Choose three to five herbs and mix them together.

Calendula: This herb offers multiple benefits, like detoxing the body, reducing inflammation, treating yeast infections, healing scar tissue, boosting immunity, and cleansing the tissues of the body. It can also give support in menstruation, easing any discomfort or pain.

Chamomile: This one is a soothing herb that brings a deep state of peace to the body. Like lavender, this herb is great for promoting relaxation and easing insomnia.

Cinnamon: This one's a kind of wonder herb. It can help support women who have heavy menstrual bleeding that's connected to uterine fibroids or endometriosis. It has also been known to help balance bleeding during menstruation.

Damiana: This herb is great for balancing our emotions, boosting libido and pleasure, and regulating the menstrual cycle.

Hibiscus: These dried flower petals work to nourish the uterine lining.

Lavender: One of my favorites. This herb promotes calm and relaxation. It de-stresses, helps combat insomnia, and reduces inflammation.

Lemon balm: This herb works wonders for de-stressing the mind and body. It also promotes emotional health and works to combat depression and anxiety.

Motherwort: This powerful herb balances hormones, eases menstrual cramps, boosts circulation, and nourishes the reproductive organs.

Peppermint: This is a great one for getting rid of infection and ridding the body of yeast from candida. It's also an energizing herb. But the thing about peppermint is, you don't want too much of it. It'll be uncomfortable for the vagina, and you might feel a stinging sensation. So, if you use peppermint, use just a little bit. If I need to use peppermint, I just take a pinch of it and toss it into my herbal mix.

Red raspberry: This one is a great herb for women. It helps bring balance to the body during menstruation so you have a normal blood flow. In general, red raspberry is excellent for nourishing and balancing the female reproductive organs. It helps tone the uterine muscles as well.

Rosemary: Another one of my favorites. The magic of this herb is its ability to get rid of yeast infections and candida. It's a blood cleanser, and it gets rid of bacteria that the body doesn't need while keeping the beneficial bacteria.

Rose petals: Not only does the fragrance of rose petals bring a tantalizing element to your yoni steam, but it offers numerous benefits. Rose petals bring relaxation, anti-inflammatory powers, a reduction of menstrual cramps, a boost in fertility, and support for a healthy digestive system. They're also steeped in sensuality and love, and they can bring about self-love and a boost in overall pleasure.

HOW TO: YONI STEAM

Once you have all your tools and herbs, it's time to get this yoni steam party started.

First, prepare the water. You don't want it to get too hot. Some people think their water has to be boiling hot in order to get the true benefits of a yoni steam. But boiling water is uncomfortable and could even burn the yoni.

The ideal temperature for a yoni steam is between 150 degrees and 160 degrees Fahrenheit. Boiling water comes in at about 180 degrees, and so you want to be sure never to sit over a pot of boiling water. And caution: I just want to make clear that you should never immerse your skin or vulvar area in this water; this is only meant to be used for steaming purposes.

If you don't have a hot plate that will show you the temperature, using the stove works just fine. Add your herbs into the pot of water. Then bring your water to a soft boil for several minutes. After that, turn off the heat and put a lid over your pot. Let your herbs steep for five minutes or so.

If you're using the hot plate, you can also add your herbs right at the start and allow them all to heat up. Try to be intentional about dropping your herbs inside your pot. Think about your intentions for using them. You might even want to silently express gratitude for the herbs you're using.

Once the water is ready, it's time to sit. Something to keep in mind: a steam should always be comfortable and feel just right. You never want to sit down over a steam and feel as if you have to breathe deeply and concentrate hard so you can bear it. If that's the case, it's way too hot. Comfort is key here, so listen to your body.

When your water is ready, you can place your hand over it to make sure it won't be too hot and uncomfortable. Then you can set it up inside your yoni throne or box or under your lawn chair. (Note that if you're using the box along with the hot plate, this makes things a lot easier. You can actually heat the hot plate and pot while they're inside the box.)

If you don't have a yoni throne or box or lawn chair, you can always make things work with a regular chair. You'll just need to sit right at the edge of it so that your yoni is exposed to the steam.

Make sure you have your gown on, or your towel over your waist. You don't want to wear any underwear or pants, as you want to completely expose your yoni to the steam. If you have a long skirt you can wear for trapping the heat, you can always use that instead of the gown.

Once you're sitting, you can start to relax. Avoid using this time for making phone calls, texting, scrolling through social media, or doing anything work related. A yoni steam is much more powerful if you're aware and present for it. Take some womb breaths, journal, meditate, reflect, and, above all, just allow yourself to deeply relax.

Again, if you can't deeply relax because you don't feel comfortable with the water temperature, that's a sign you need to turn down the heat or—if your pot isn't on a hot plate—wait until the temperature drops a bit. A yoni steam requires a fully relaxed state of surrender to the process.

Steam for about forty-five minutes, or sixty minutes max, if you're feeling it and want to keep going. It might be tempting to go longer, but you don't want to overdo it.

THE PERFECT TIME TO STEAM

Never do a yoni steam while you're on your period or if you're pregnant. The best time to do a yoni steam is after menstruation. That way, you can help your body release any other remaining residue or energy that didn't get released during your period. It's a great way of allowing your body a chance to deeply reset and clear the board before you continue your cycle and prepare for ovulation.

If you're trying to get pregnant, only steam during the window between menstruation and ovulation. Definitely don't steam after ovulation; wait until you've menstruated and have the confirmation that you're not pregnant.

MEDITATIONS FOR YONI STEAMING

While you're steaming your yoni, you can also use some basic meditations to guide you in being more present to the process. Being present, open, and available during your steam will put you in a calmer, more receptive frame of mind. It might even stir up some deep insights, wisdom, visions, and creative ideas inside of you. Be sure to keep a journal next to you in case you need to quickly jot something down.

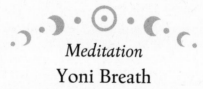

Meditation

Sensations of Yoni Steaming

Once you're sitting down over your yoni steam throne, start to take some womb breaths. Allow yourself to be completely present to the sensation of the steam and the herbs entering your yoni. Give yourself over to the feeling of the warmth touching your body. Feel it moving into your yoni. Trust that it will do exactly what it needs to do to bring you into a whole, balanced, peaceful, healthy, and joyful state. Don't forget to keep breathing deeply as you do this. You can do this basic yoni steam meditation for as long as you like. If any insights or revelations drop into your mind, don't forget to write them down.

Meditation

Yoni Breath

As you're receiving your yoni steam, take a few deep womb breaths. Now, concentrate your energy at the opening of your yoni. Keep your attention there, and just feel all the sensation. Focus so deeply on the opening of your yoni that it's as if you become this part of yourself, and everything else around you melts away.

After a few minutes of concentrating here, imagine you are taking your next inhale straight down into the opening of your yoni. And when you exhale, feel the opening of your yoni soften and relax. Do this for at least five minutes.

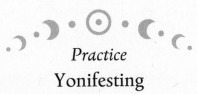

Meditation

Breasts and Yoni Steam

During this meditation, you'll be visualizing the herbs and steam moving up into your breasts and heart, and then you'll move that energy back down and out.

This will bring the energy from your breasts into your womb and yoni and help cleanse and purify the heart area.

As you receive your yoni steam, center yourself by taking a few deep womb breaths.

When you're ready, as you inhale through the nose, imagine you are pulling the steam through your yoni and all the way up into both your breasts. Hold that energy here for a few seconds, just allowing the herbal mixture and steam to settle deep into your breasts. Then, exhale through the mouth, and imagine you are moving the steam and herbs down from your breasts, through the womb, out the yoni, and back into the pot.

Continue repeating this visualization for five to ten minutes. The important thing with this one is that you take your time with it. There's nowhere to go, nowhere to rush to, and nothing as important as this moment right here. Slow down and let yourself drop into the moment.

Practice

Yonifesting

While you're doing your yoni steam, it's a great opportunity to manifest and start envisioning all you'd like to create in your life. Every herb carries a different energy, and many are great for manifesting.

You can pick your herbs based on what you desire and want to call in to your life.

Here's a list of some of my favorite herbs for manifesting...

Basil: For abundance, money, protection
Bay leaf: For psychic powers, protection
Cinnamon: For prosperity, success
Clove: For love, money
Jasmine: For soul mate attraction
Lavender: For happiness, peace, harmony
Marjoram: For attracting wealth, drawing love to you
Mint: For protection, money
Rose petals: For deep friendships, domestic peace, divine love

Once you've gotten your manifesting herbs into the mix, receive your yoni steam and breathe deeply as you visualize all the things you'd like to manifest.

Your manifesting abilities are super heightened when you can actually start to *feel* the thing you're manifesting. This doesn't just apply to when you're doing a yoni steam, but during any other time you're working to manifest and create.

A visualization without feeling is like going back in time and watching television in black and white. Your visualization will take on an empty, hollow feeling, and it will be disconnected from you. If you can't feel it, you can't manifest it.

If you're seeking a romantic partner but all you feel inside is lonely and frustrated, that's all you're going to get. However, if you're seeking a romantic partner and you can hone in on a feeling of deep, blooming love and compassion within you, then you've got something. You've cultivated something within you that is going to have a magnetic charge and help you manifest.

So, as you steam your yoni, give yourself over to the feeling of what you want.

If you can feel it, you can create it.

Start by seeing what you want in your mind, and then allow your body to feel as if this thing you're seeing is really happening in your life right this second. Feel that excitement, that sense of joy, that sense of wholeness, in your body right now. Don't wait until you've actually acquired the thing. We waste too much time aspiring, yearning, and pining for things, and not enough time just feeling the way we want to *right now*.

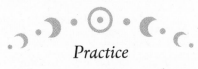

Practice
Yoni Steam Journaling

As you do your yoni steam, you can even set aside some time to do a journaling practice. Pull out your journal and allow yourself to empty all your thoughts onto the paper. Stay relaxed and present, and let the yoni steam bring you into an open state. Write down any ideas, visions, or feelings that might arise in the moment. Combining womb magic with herbal magic makes for a potent mix, so be aware of all that is coming up within your mind, heart, and body.

WHAT TO EXPECT AFTER A YONI STEAM

After your yoni steam is completed, be gentle with yourself for the rest of the day. Be sure to go slow and to listen to your inner voice. Do only what feels good to you.

Ideally, you won't have to go to work or do something physically grueling after a yoni steam. To truly allow the experience to integrate, make sure to take care of yourself and let yourself be guided by what your body needs.

You might notice that your body is more relaxed and at ease and that you sleep better at night after your steam! Dreams may appear more vividly, and you might even find yourself experiencing a true state of wellness, joy, and connectedness to your body and spirit.

Be sure to drink a lot of water in the days that follow your yoni steam so that you can help push out any remaining energies that need to be released.

How Often?

Once you start doing yoni steams, you might be tempted to start doing them all the time. Some people recommend a good yoni steam every other day, or every week. One to three times a month is ideal.

However, if you have an issue you're working to treat, you might want to aim for at least once a week for a couple of months.

I stick to doing a steam once a month a couple of days after my period to help my body cleanse and release anything that did not leave during menstruation. If you don't have a period, you can do a steam during the part of the month that feels best for you. Around the time of the new moon is ideal since it's the start of another cycle. Doing your yoni steam around the new moon will help put you in sync with nature and wipe the slate clean by cleansing your womb and allowing you to start anew.

Chapter 9 Takeaways

- Steaming isn't about cleaning the womb and vagina. It goes way deeper than that. It's a healing, restorative self-care practice.
- Yoni steaming can regulate menstruation, boost fertility, heal the womb of any imbalances, detoxify the body, promote relaxation, nourish the reproductive organs, enhance immunity, deepen pleasure, and improve digestion.
- A yoni steam can be done comfortably at home with a pot, towel or gown, herbs, appropriate chair, and water.
- During your yoni steam, be fully present. You'll get the most benefits this way. Focus on how your body feels as the steam enters you. Do meditations, visualizations, and journaling to immerse yourself more deeply in the process.

Chapter 10

MENSTRUATION

"The menstrual cycle governs the feminine flow, not only of each monthly bleed, but also of information, emotions, spirituality and creativity."
—Lisa Lister[21]

> **NOTE:** If you're a woman who doesn't menstruate, you can still take advantage of the power inherent in the menstrual cycle. You can, instead, work with the rhythm of the moon. The moon is on a 29.5-day cycle, which is very close to the average 28-day menstrual cycle.

When I was younger, my period was enemy number one.

It always seemed to rear its head at the most inopportune times—vacations, birthday parties, weekend excursions. It was like my period, somehow, always knew when I was about to do something fun.

I'd be excitedly getting on a plane, ready to head off on a trip, and then—my period would start. Even on the night of my wedding, when I was excited to finally be alone with my husband and have some intimate time together—my period suddenly started. It was seriously like a thorn in my side, always magically appearing at the worst times to interrupt and deter me.

"I hate my period," I often found myself saying. It was like a mantra for me.

---

21. Lisa Lister, *Love Your Lady Landscape* (London: Hay House, 2016), 84.

Every single time it came around, I would chant this like my life depended on it. Like saying these words would somehow fix things.

To me, getting my period was the ultimate hinderance and inconvenience. It was "cramping my style," leaving me unable to do as I pleased.

During my days of heavy flow, there was this feeling in my body, this voice that told me to sit back and allow myself some rest. But I wasn't having any of that. Since I was always on the go, it annoyed me to have to slow down. The only thing I could think to do was to keep trying to push myself, as if everything was business as usual. In doing so, I'd show my period who was boss.

After years of operating this way, things started to change.

I started to learn more about my body, my womb, the moon, cycles, and feminine energy. I started to explore and understand just how sacred and precious menstruation really was. The realization of this hit me so hard, and I couldn't help but regret all the time I had spent despising the one thing that encompassed ... *everything*.

I never imagined I would be someone who would literally jump up and down with excitement when I realized my period was starting.

Now, instead of "I hate my period," I eagerly proclaim to anyone within earshot, "I got my period!" It's something I celebrate every single time. And that sense of celebration allows me to embrace my womb and who I am as a woman, more deeply than I ever have before.

If you're still currently menstruating, don't let the opportunity pass you by. Each cycle is a precious chance to go inside, to reconnect and reclaim your power as a woman.

Your bleed is one of the highest forms of creative expression your body can make.

It's a time to realign to the creativity, beauty, and magic that you are. Every part of the cycle is a time for this, but the bleeding part of it, especially so. It's the time when blood, as well as some tissue, from inside of your womb are moving outside of your body. Since the womb is a source of power, anything that flows from it is also coursing with that same power.

Your Blood Is Sacred

After I graduated from college, I moved to Los Angeles with my boyfriend, trying to find work as an actress while balancing a ton of odd jobs. I did a lot of background extra work in movies and TV shows. You'd basically have to watch them without blinking, because then you'd miss seeing me entirely. I also had a ton of starring roles in music videos, short films, B movies, commercials, and independent films—you name it, I've done it.

The year before leaving college in Boston, I was nineteen. Since I knew I was moving to Los Angeles to pursue becoming an actress, I wanted to get all the experience I could. So, I acted in a bunch of different student films. During this one production, I remember shooting a romantic scene with some actor I had just met about thirty minutes prior to filming. It wasn't anything serious. There was no kissing or nudity. I think we were just lying on a bed together and cuddling.

Between takes, the actor asked me if I had a boyfriend. I told him I did, but he continued to hit on me every time the camera stopped running, asking more and more questions, and being incredibly attentive to everything I was saying.

At the time, I was on day two of my period. The heaviest flow day for me.

I was experiencing some menstrual cramps between takes, and I happened to mention this to the guy I was acting with.

You would've thought I had said the most vile, disgusting thing of all time, because the guy looked as if he were about to throw up.

"You're on your period?" he whispered.

I nodded, not really understanding what the big deal was.

He backed up, about a couple of feet away from me. And for the rest of the time we shot that scene, he was cold and detached. He couldn't look me in the eye or talk to me for the rest of the day.

Part of me was happy, because at least he was leaving me alone; but the other part of me felt like I had done something wrong. *Maybe I shouldn't have said anything; or worse, maybe I shouldn't have even shown up to do the film shoot, because a woman on her period is gross and shouldn't be around other people.*

After that, I made a mental note to never again mention to anyone that I was on my period.

Many girls and women have gone through the feeling of being shamed during their periods. Somehow, this myth that it's a dirty thing that shouldn't really be discussed has been perpetuated. And so, we fall in line, speaking of our period in low tones, if we speak about it at all.

In certain areas of countries like Nepal and India, women are separated from their villages if they're on their period, as they're considered impure and unfit to engage in normal society. They're made to live out in huts that are oftentimes unsanitary and unsafe.[22] During the time of the month when they should be luxuriating in their inner queendom, they're cast aside, as if something is inherently wrong with them.

Having our periods isn't something dirty or shameful.
It's a natural and beautiful part of who we are.

Science tells us that our menstrual blood contains all kinds of benefits. Studies have been done to show that our menstrual blood contains stem cells, as well as therapeutic and antibacterial properties.[23] Some women have even taken to saving their menstrual blood and using it to make face masks, swearing by its ability to keep their skin nice and clear. Menstrual blood is also known to work as a great fertilizer for growing plants and trees.

22. "Chhaupadi and menstruation taboos," Action Aid, last modified May 23, 2022, https://www.actionaid.org.uk/our-work/period-poverty/chhaupadi-and-menstruation-taboos.

23. Lijun Chen, Jingjing Qu, Tianli Cheng, Xin Chen, and Charlie Xiang, "Menstrual blood-derived stem cells: toward therapeutic mechanisms, novel strategies, and future perspectives in the treatment of diseases," *Stem Cell Research & Therapy* 10 (December 2019): 406, https://stemcellres.biomedcentral.com/articles/10.1186/s13287-019-1503-7; Pawel Mak, Kinga Wojcik, Lukasz Wicherek, Piotr Suder, and Adam Dubin, "Antibacterial hemoglobin peptides in human menstrual blood," Peptides 25, no. 11 (November 2004): 1839–1847, https://pubmed.ncbi.nlm.nih.gov/15501514/.

This womb blood is overflowing with all kinds of powerful properties that science is just beginning to understand and take note of. Hopefully, over time, this will help reduce the stigma that still lingers out there surrounding menstruation. As you bleed each month, remember that the blood that flows from you contains power and potential.

Understanding the magic of menstruation is a big part of nurturing wellness for your womb. The blood that flows from us is steeped in power. And the understanding of its sacredness has been lost over time, which has weakened women's connection to their body and womb.

Why Is Menstruation So Powerful?

Every month, the intelligence of a woman's body naturally delves into the work of preparing for pregnancy. During menstruation, blood sheds from the womb, down the cervix, and out of the vagina. There are four phases to this miraculous cycle that our bodies naturally navigate without us having to give it all a single thought.

Our lack of alignment to and appreciation for our menstrual cycle can sometimes lead to uncomfortable cramps, fatigue, pain, irritability, and headaches. If you're someone who struggles with these kinds of symptoms, try to be more conscious of your body and your cycle. You might notice that things will start to shift, and these kinds of symptoms might lessen or completely dissipate. Love and honor the brilliance that is your body, and you will start to feel a deep sense of coming back home to yourself.

Phase 1: Menses Phase

During this phase, which marks the beginning of the cycle, the uterus's lining sheds from the vagina, if there's no pregnancy. The bleeding lasts for about three to five days.

At this time, a woman is in her true power. As this blood flows from your womb, your body is able to clear and release all the things from the last cycle you need to let go of. Being conscious of surrendering to this process of letting go is key. This will help you clear yourself more quickly of any residue left behind from challenging experiences, emotions, and feelings from your last cycle.

During your lifetime, your womb absorbs the things you feel and experience. If something within you needs to be released, your menses phase is the time to do this. It's the ultimate form of release. Practice self-care during this time, and give yourself the opportunity to slow down and let your body feel this experience. Some of us just want our periods to be over as soon as possible, so we can get on to the next thing. I hear you; I've been there. But if you can start slowing down, and being conscious of surrendering to your period, you can summon all your creative powers and energies.

As the blood moves out of your body, you can claim it as something other than an inconvenience or annoyance. You can take the time to acknowledge your power and magic as a woman on this planet. You can honor yourself for the beauty and life-giving potential you naturally hold. You can wrap your arms around yourself in celebration. Give yourself a deep hug as you breathe and feel the power you carry.

Don't ever forget the magic that you are.
Don't ever let the routine of life lull you into believing
you are something other than a miracle.

Your blood, as it flows, is a reminder of your power. Don't fall asleep and succumb to the lie that you're not good enough, that you can't do this or that, that you'll never fulfill all the desires bursting in your heart.

Bring yourself back through awareness. Let your womb, your menstrual cycle, guide you back to yourself, back to the wild and untamed woman you truly are.

During your bleed, create what you can, if it feels right. Paint, sing, draw, write, sculpt, shape, transform. Use your hands and your heart. Journal about all visions calling to you. Dare yourself to reimagine your life during this new cycle that is starting. Fall asleep and dream of your ancestors, of all the ones who came before you, of the ones who made it possible for you to be here.

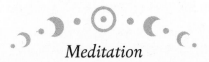

Meditation
Menstruation Mindfulness

While you're bleeding, especially during the heavy days, try to do some meditation. This will help you surrender more deeply to the process of releasing, allowing your blood to flow, and clearing your energies.

Drape yourself in something red, like a scarf or a blanket. Since the red color symbolizes your blood, it will help bring you into a place of deeper consciousness and awareness for your period.

Sit or lie down—whatever is most comfortable for you. Listen to your body to find out how it wants to be positioned, and it will tell you.

When you're ready, place both hands over your womb. Start to breathe deeply through the nose, and just notice what's happening within your womb. Feel the sacred process of menstruation dancing within you and moving outward. Just notice what's happening. Breathe and connect with the magic that is occurring. Give it your full awareness as you continue to breathe. Let your breath be a soothing balm to the insides of your body and womb as you continue to stay aware. Try to do this for about five to ten minutes.

This meditation can be done as often as you like, throughout your period. It's a way of honoring your body for the miraculous work it's undertaking. This meditation will give you a chance to slow down, be gentle with yourself, and practice self-care. Being aware as your blood moves out of you is a very gentle process that aligns you to your feminine gifts of flow and surrender.

Mindfulness during menstruation gives us the opportunity to relax into ourselves; not to strain or strive for anything more, but to exist in the simple space of being.

MENSTRUATION IS MAGIC

Menstruation's magic happens without our conscious input, just like with breathing. Our bodies know how to breathe without any effort on our part, and so we take our breathing for granted and don't pay it any mind at all.

We've taken the power of menstruation for granted long enough.

What if we made menstruation into an intentional process of self-care, release, discovery, and power harnessing? So that instead of feeling annoyed or inconvenienced or bothered by it, we feel empowered by it?

It becomes like that feeling of excitement that happens when a cherished friend visits our home. Eager for warmth, connection, and conversation with this friend, we make sure that everything is just right. Before she arrives, our minds pay attention to things we probably wouldn't have noticed before. We straighten up a bit and prepare for the encounter.

When she arrives, we're attentive to what she might need—a drink, a snack, the bathroom. We devote our focus and our energy to this friend, grateful for the time we have with her.

Do this, also, with your period. Let it be your best friend. Love it, nurture it, melt into it. Become addicted to knowing it more intimately than you thought was humanely possible.

Your period is your power.

Own the experience of menstruation. Relish every moment. Even if you're feeling crampy, or tired, or uninterested in being social. Sit with that and accept it. Don't force something that's not there.

Your power lies in your ability to feel what's present, not to ignore what's inside of you. Strength is centered around acknowledging and feeling your emotions, whereas weakness is based upon pretending to feel something other than what you really do feel.

Denying what's inside of you is self-betrayal. And when you betray the self, it's hard to love and care for the self.

Self-care and *self-love* are big buzzwords lately that everybody seems to be talking about—which is a good thing. But don't settle. Don't skate on the surface of what you think self-care and self-love should look like. Go deeper. Know who you are inside, and honor that. Honor your menstruation. You only get so many cycles, so many opportunities, to embrace what is your inherent power.

PHASE 2: FOLLICULAR PHASE

The next part of the menstrual cycle is the follicular phase. This phase usually happens from day six to day fourteen. Estrogen rises in your body, causing the lining of your uterus to thicken. In your ovaries, follicles start to grow and develop. At the end of this phase, a fully mature egg will develop from one of the follicles.

During the follicular phase, your body is undergoing the work of creating the potential for life. This is a time for opportunity, creativity, and expansion. Your energy will be high, which makes this a good time to drive projects, goals, and visions forward. Your womb has just cleared itself, releasing energies that were with you from the last cycle. Now that the process is finished, you might notice a very grounded yet expansive feeling within you. Your ability to get things done is greater than normal, so be intentional about what you'd like to accomplish during this time.

Movement is suggested during the follicular phase. After your period is finished, you might notice that your body naturally craves physical movement and action. Carve out some time to do things, like hiking, stretching, yoga, and dance. Allow your body to be free. Find ways to let it express itself. Our bodies sometimes get stuck in moving in the same patterns due to our daily routines. Look for opportunities to switch up the habitual ways your body is accustomed to, and do something that might be a little different.

When we move differently, we're opening up new pathways in our brains, as well as in our energy channels. This can affect us mentally and emotionally and create more ways of processing, releasing, and understanding what's happening around us and within us.

Practice
Shake It Out

Shaking is a good way of releasing energy, freeing your body, and breaking up any patterns of habitual movements. Not only is it fun, but it's quite simple to do.

Play some upbeat music. Try to find something without words so that you can offer your fullest attention. This shaking exercise works best if you allow your mind to take a back seat. If there are words in the song, your mind may be tempted to listen to them or sing along.

Keep your feet planted on the ground and close your eyes.

Shake out every part of your body. Just allow yourself to release and fully let go. Don't forget to breathe.

If any thoughts come up in the mind, just imagine you're shaking your thoughts right out, and keep going.

Try to shake for at least fifteen to twenty minutes.

Shaking is an effective way of aligning yourself to the present moment. It's a form of movement meditation you can use whenever you need, even just for a quick two- to three-minute session.

PHASE 3: OVULATION

At about fourteen days into your cycle, ovulation occurs, allowing for the ovary to release its egg after an increase in the luteinizing hormone and the follicle-stimulating hormone. During this part of the cycle, your mental and creative energies are at an all-time high. This is a time when new, exciting ideas might be sparked, and a boost to your mental capacity will help you hone your focus and dig in to figuring things out.

With estrogen levels rising during this time, the activity in the left hemisphere is also enhanced. This means that verbal fluency is greater during ovulation, which is something all of us can take advantage of. You'll be able to "find the words" and communicate with more ease and clarity during this time. If there are any important conversations you need to have, or people you want to cultivate deeper connections with, make a point to interact during this phase in the cycle. It's also a good time for public speaking, making presentations, and asking for what you want.

During ovulation, studies have also shown that our libido is a lot higher. Pheromones are released by our bodies, boosting our sexual attractiveness to others. Knowing this, you can use that enhanced sexual energy to fuel your current relationship, or if you don't have a partner and would like one, you can even direct this energy toward finding a new relationship.

Our sexual energy is our vitality and life force energy. Its vibrant force is what birthed us into being, and its energy continues to sustain us each and every single day. It's what animates our bodies, our wombs, and our hearts.

Our society has a very limited definition of what sex and sexuality really are. And so, we've built up so much guilt and shame surrounding them, which has led to a disconnect from our bodies and from loving who we are. During ovulation, it's empowering to own your sexuality and to bask in the energy of its sacredness.

The period of ovulation offers a tiny window of time, lasting only twenty-four hours. So, if you know you're in the ovulation phase, take advantage of the fleeting opportunity by doing some practices to increase your connection to your sexual energy.

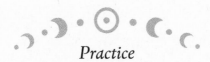

Practice

Harness Your Sexual Energy

This is a great practice to do during ovulation or any other time you feel you need a boost in sexual energy.

Sit comfortably in a chair, or cross-legged on the floor.

Close your eyes and take a few womb breaths here.

Now, focus on the opening of your vagina. Allow yourself to melt into the opening, to really feel your body melting into the vagina. Give it your focus and attention as you continue to breathe deeply.

After a few minutes, imagine a beautiful flower sitting in your vagina. When you inhale, feel the petals of that flower and your vagina open together; when you exhale, feel the petals of the flower and your vagina close. Do this for a few minutes.

Now just breathe normally and let go of the visualization.

Allow yourself to take a minute to scan your body. See if you notice anything new, like a kind of vitality seeping into your cells. If you don't notice anything, this is perfectly okay. Chances are, there are sensations happening at a very subtle level in the body. But if you're just starting to go on this journey, you might not notice all these feelings yet.

Commit to doing this exercise at least once a month during ovulation time. You can also try this exercise during any other parts of the month, whether you're ovulating or not. The more you do this, the more you will start to notice shifts within you.

Trust your unique journey, and know you're always exactly where you need to be.

Phase 4: Luteal Phase

The luteal phase happens from about day fifteen to day twenty-eight. In this phase, the egg moves through the fallopian tubes and over to the womb. Progesterone rises to help prep the lining of the uterus for a possible pregnancy.

During this phase, it's time to start slowing down and tuning in. This is a time for being aware of our needs and listening to our bodies. Focus your energies inward and release any attachments and expectations.

Drink a lot of water during this phase, and allow yourself to be in a flowing, receptive state. In this phase, your body has the ability to notice things you might not normally notice during the month, and your intuition might be sharper than usual.

Try not to resist the flow of intuition, insights, and revelations that might be sparking within you. When we resist the flow of intuition, this can allow for PMS to pop up, bringing us discomfort and a feeling that we're not in control of our emotions and bodies.

The luteal phase is your opportunity to really sit with who you are and to allow your inner wisdom to shine through. It's a time of understanding what things you need to release in order to be your truest self.

Journal about how you feel, practice self-massage, go for walks out in nature, find time for stillness, and listen to your body as much as you can. The awareness that you put into your luteal phase will help bring about a smoother menstruation. It will ease your body naturally into the process. If you're dealing with any challenging PMS symptoms, being aware and slowing down during your luteal phase will help you feel more balanced.

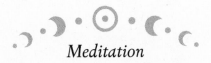

Meditation
Luteal Phase Mindfulness

For this meditation, find a comfortable spot where you can lie down without interruptions.

Get into a fetal position, as if you were back in the womb. Bring your knees up toward your forehead, as much as you can. If any of this is uncomfortable, make adjustments to ensure your body feels good. Wrap your arms around your knees if you're able to do so.

In this position, allow all the muscles in your body to relax. Start to take deep womb breaths. Let yourself stay this way for as long as you need to. Try to let your mind be still. However, if any thoughts come up, don't get discouraged. Notice them, and then come back to the present moment, to the breath and to the body.

OWN EACH PHASE

Each phase comes with its own magic, offering you a chance to realign to your feminine gifts, energies, and powers. Connecting to your own menstrual cycle puts you in lockstep with nature, so that you are forming a bridge between yourself and all cycles that currently exist.

Is there anything more powerful than that?

Give yourself over to the intelligence of your flow, to the natural cycle that is always working through you. Honoring yourself in this way is effortless, yet radically life changing.

UNDERSTANDING YOUR OWN UNIQUE CYCLE

Understanding how your menstrual cycle unfolds will offer you some clues and insights on how your energy and moods shift over the course of several weeks. One of the ways to do this is by tracking it.

When I was a teenager, and during most of my twenties, I didn't bother with tracking or paying any mind to what my cycle looked like. 'Cause I didn't really care. I didn't want my period to happen at all, and so tracking wasn't a priority for me.

When I started gaining more wisdom about the beauty of menstruation, I began to track my cycle. And I discovered so many things about how my mindset, moods, and energy levels changed according to where I was at in my cycle.

Understanding how your cycle impacts you can give you the clarity to really know what you need as you go about your week.

For instance, if you know you always tend to feel low in energy and unmotivated in the days leading up to your period, you'll know not to plan to work on certain projects that might require a ton of focus. If you know you have the greatest amount of energy after your period, you can plan for all the outings and projects that require you to be high energy.

Tracking puts you in a strong position. It helps you cultivate an inner awareness of what's transpiring in your mind, body, heart, and spirit.

The first month of tracking is the discovery month. It's all about going through each day of your cycle, and at the end of the day, jotting down a few words about anything you noticed in terms of how you felt—mentally, physically, emotionally, and spiritually. Since many of us don't often make time to check in with ourselves, it's a great way of developing awareness for what's happening inside of you throughout your cycle.

After you get a sense of your first month, go in and track the second month to see if your moods and energies are pretty consistent with the last month. If they are, you pretty much have an understanding of what your regular rhythms are throughout the cycle. If they're not consistent, try to do a third month of tracking, and look for overlap there.

If you still don't notice any patterns, not to worry. You might not find any consistency in your natural feminine rhythms. Sometimes we become out of sync with our bodies, but all it takes is a little awareness to get back on track. If you're having trouble finding patterns, go deeper. Become more acutely aware of what your body is trying to express to you. Slow down and listen, and you will hear its inner rhythms. You will understand exactly what it needs. Nurturing a deeper sense of awareness of your body will bring you into a state of ease and inner clarity. Along with the body, there is another way to realign—and it involves using the energy of the moon as your anchor.

THE MOON AND MENSTRUATION

The energy that women hold is deeply intertwined with that of the moon. The moon, with its natural power and grace, controls the ocean tides. It's very much linked with and connected to water, just as the womb is.

Throughout time, many have speculated and written about women's connection with the glowing ball of lunar light in the sky. This is based on the fact that both women's menstrual cycle and the moon's lunar cycle roughly last for the same amount of time. A moon cycle goes for 29.5 days, while a woman's menstrual cycle comes in at between 25 and 30 days.

Along with the moon, we see cycles at work all around us. The earth would cease to exist if cycles suddenly came to a halt. Our planet depends on the dynamic power of cycles as it constantly shifts and evolves over time. The water cycle, carbon cycle, rock cycle, and nitrogen cycle all sustain us and our world. Seasons move through cycles, as do the sun and all the planets in our galaxy. Nothing is static in this ever-changing world. Nature depends on the consistency of cycles to keep moving forward and generating new life.

It makes sense, then, that we, as women, carry the power of cycles within us. This is what charges our connection to Mother Nature. Our bodies contain the miraculous ability to create life. Without the power of cycles that is deeply embedded in our wombs and feminine systems, we'd have no way to do this.

Over time, we've lost touch with our natural cycles. In a recent study on the connection between menstruation and the moon, scientists hypothesized that our changing lifestyles and exposure to artificial light might have driven many of us to fall out of step with the lunar cycle.[24]

As I've come to experience: we're all different, and we shouldn't feel like our bodies aren't doing what they should be doing just because our periods don't start with the new moon. Our bodies have their own intuition and wisdom and work in ways that are conducive to what we truly need.

If you're a woman who doesn't menstruate, you can use the moon cycle to track your moods and feelings. Carve out some time to sit outside under the moon and meditate on it. Feel the ways in which your own energy integrates with the energy inherent in the moon. Imagine yourself sitting in the center of the moon and let your every pore drink in its healing, rejuvenating powers. And you can also do all this even if you do menstruate. Sitting with the moon provides us with a tangible way of falling back in sync with nature, cycles, and our feminine energies.

USING MENSTRUATION TO MANIFEST

Since menstruation brings women to the full height of their power, it's a great time for manifesting your dreams and desires. The powers of creation are running through you, setting the stage for you to vision and manifest, should you so desire. Manifestation is a way of bringing your intentions, goals, and desires all out onto the physical plane.

Manifestation is a process of setting intentions, visualizing, embodying, and taking the necessary action to make things happen. Sometimes it's easy

---

24. Maria Cohut, "Menstrual Cycles and Lunar Cycles: Is There a Link?" Medical News Today, February 12, 2021, https://www.medicalnewstoday.com/articles/menstrual-cycles-and-lunar-cycles-is-there-a-link.

to lose sight of the fact that action is an essential part of the process. It's simple to write down some goals, or pray, or light a candle—and then move on and forget, thinking we've already done what's required.

But manifestation goes beyond the visualizing and intention setting. It has to be felt inside the body, and that feeling has to be taken and transmuted into tangible action. So, we're not just sitting around, waiting for things to happen to us. We're employing some of that inner will and taking the required actions to propel our lives forward.

The heart of manifestation is hinged upon *alignment*. It's about aligning to who you are within, and liberating all the sensual, creative, dynamic, vibrant forces inside of you. Once you do this, you naturally become more magnetic. That magnetism is going to attract exactly what you need to you, without you even having to devote a conscious thought to it. This is an advanced way to manifest—trusting that the universe is working with you and will bring you exactly what you need in the moment you need it. Having this kind of trust is wildly freeing and releases our need to control or pour energy into dictating how every little detail in our lives is going to go.

The universe is always working with you.

Owning your menstrual cycle, surrendering to the power of your womb and your own inner magic, will help awaken your ultimate manifesting potential. This doesn't mean that once you awaken all your feminine powers and gifts there will be no more pain, loss, or challenges in your life. We'll still experience some rough patches here and there. Our souls are on this planet to learn, evolve, and grow. Without the darkness, there can be no light. Our challenges mold who we are, build our character, make us stronger in the face of fear. Look at your life challenges as your hidden blessings, your opportunities to grow and enhance all that you are.

Aligning to your menstrual cycle, or the moon cycle, is a way of manifesting exactly what you need when you need it. By surrendering to your cycle, your body, and your womb, you are giving yourself over to the infinite intelligence that permeates this universe. That infinite intelligence, that *source*, is something we're always connected to, even if we're not conscious of it.

Embrace the power of the cycles within your gorgeous body. That is true manifestation. That is the path to your deepest power.

CHAPTER 10 TAKEAWAYS

- Your period is a natural part of who you are, not something to be ashamed of.
- Your power is inherent in your bleed. The blood that flows from you is an expression of all the wisdom, beauty, and life-giving energy you contain as a woman.
- Becoming more mindful of your cycle will help you stay balanced.
- Track your cycle to get clarity around the way your mood, energy levels, and feelings shift throughout the month.
- Meditate with the moon to align yourself to the power of nature and cycles.
- Owning the power of your menstrual cycle naturally makes you better at manifesting and creating the life you want.

Chapter 11

MENOPAUSE

"If you want to know where your power really is, you need look no further than the processes of your body that you've been taught to dismiss, deny, or be afraid of. These include the menstrual cycle, labor, and, the mother of all wake-up calls, menopause."

—Christiane Northrup, MD[25]

With every year that passes, I become less and less concerned with what people think of me. When I was younger, I used to feel this pressure of trying to live up to others' expectations of what I should do and be in my life. But as time went on, I realized how foolish that was. I started to relax into myself, to trust the ways in which I wanted to show up in the world.

As women age, we step more fully into our wisdom. And menopause plays a great part in bringing us into that transition, allowing us to embody our older, wiser selves.

Although I haven't personally experienced menopause yet, I felt it was important to include in this book. I've been reading up on it and taking in everything I can from other women's experiences to prepare myself for the shifts ahead. I believe it's important to discuss and acknowledge this very unique and potent time in a woman's life.

---

25. Christiane Northrup, *Women's Bodies, Women's Wisdom*, 5th ed. (New York: Bantam Books, 2020), 638.

Menopause is a time of transformation. It's a shift toward a new way of being and living in your unique feminine body. Some of us might look at this time as a difficult period in which we are closing the door on our youth and steering into the time of old age. We might feel as if we've lost some of our magic, as we no longer bleed and hold that same connection to our wombs.

But all of that is simply untrue. Even though menopause carries us away from menstruation, signifying our inability to birth children, this doesn't mean our power as women is lost to us.

In actuality, our power is being refined. For as we age, as we evolve and transform, we become more able to channel wisdom, truth, and love. We become equipped to traverse into the greater depths of our beings. This gives us the ability to show up fully as ourselves, no apologies needed.

Menopause carries great possibility. However, it might not seem like it when your hormone levels are changing and your body is experiencing a myriad of chaotic shifts. As you're going through menopause, you might start to feel disappointed, as if your body is failing you. *But it's not.*

Menopause is a time of deep transformation. It's a time for women to step into the limitlessness of their potential.

You don't need your bleed to connect you to nature and to the moon, because you're already connected. Nature's lush energies permeate within your cells. The whispers of the moon ebb and flow within the space of each breath you take. You are simply tapped in. Your womb becomes an open, clear, and radiant portal through which anything is possible. After years of bleeding, you've moved into a new phase of your life. A time in which you are fully in the driver's seat when it comes to all your emotions, feelings, thoughts, and actions.

Nothing is more powerful than a woman who braves her way through menopause and comes out on the other end. It might seem like a drag to endure something of this magnitude. It might sometimes feel like a challenge to be in this feminine form. But know that you were made to navigate this. Everything that occurs within your feminine body carries a natural rhythm, one that every cell of your being is familiar with. Things like menstruation, pregnancy, childbirth, and menopause might seem to carry countless changes and challenges, but remember, they also carry invaluable gifts that have the power to impact your life in the most profound ways.

Protect your energy, and do things that feel good to you. Allow the natural process of menopause to work its magic.

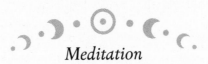

Meditation
Menopause Mindfulness

During menopause, try to use this meditation to find stillness within your body and mind. It will help you navigate this time and stay aligned to yourself.

Sit up straight and take some womb breaths.

Place your hands below your belly button, over your womb. Continue to breathe deeply here.

Imagine you are inside of your uterus. Feel what it's like to be in this space. Feel the energy, the texture, the sensation in your womb. Notice anything that might seem stuck, heavy, or uncomfortable. If you do notice anything like this, breathe into that one spot, allowing your exhale to melt away any tension that might be lingering there. Complete this until you feel as if the tension has broken up.

Go through your womb again and feel where there might be any other areas of discomfort. Repeat the same breathing process once you find any.

If you don't find any areas of discomfort, simply stay focused on the center of your womb and breathe. Be fully present and open to this space and all the magic that exists within it. Know that your body is a miracle and that the work it does to keep your system running smoothly is a sacred process.

At the end of this meditation, wrap your arms around yourself and give yourself a big hug. You *so* got this.

Meditation
Ovary Mindfulness

During menopause, the ovaries, which have been making eggs for many years, begin the process of shutting down production. This is no easy shift. It will take time and will bring about major changes to the body. The ovaries have been dedicated to this task for so long, and now they will finally be getting rest. It's an exciting time for your ovaries, and one that can feel less rocky if you're able to allow the process to happen consciously and with intention.

This meditation will help you connect with your ovaries and support them in facing the change they're enduring.

Find somewhere to lie down. Place a pillow or bolster under your knees to make yourself comfortable.

Place your left hand over the left side of your lower belly, and your right hand over the right side of your lower belly, allowing each hand to be placed on top of an ovary.

Start to take some womb breaths to activate this region.

Now, focus on the left ovary under your left hand. As you inhale through the nose, imagine your left ovary is the one taking the inhale.

And now, as you focus on the right ovary under your right hand, imagine the right ovary is exhaling the breath out.

Again: inhale through the left ovary, exhale through the right ovary. Keep this breath going for at least ten minutes. Allow yourself to truly surrender to the meditation, and really stay focused on breathing from your ovaries.

If you get distracted, come back to your ovaries under your hands, and just continue. At the end of this meditation, take a moment to feel gratitude for your ovaries and all the work they have done during your lifetime.

Chapter 11 Takeaways

- Menopause isn't a transition to fear. It's a time of transformation and power. It's an opportunity for women to come into their full wisdom.

- Losing the ability to menstruate doesn't mean you're no longer tapped into the power inherent in nature and cycles. Going through menopause brings you closer to your natural and vital self and allows you to align effortlessly to nature. It gives you a chance to uncover your rawest, most authentic, and wisest self.

- Take time to care for and listen to your body during menopause. The more you can slow down and stay connected to your body, the less rocky this time in your life will be.

Part III

HARNESSING YOUR SEXUAL ENERGY

Chapter 12

SEXUAL ENERGY AND HEALING

"Our sexual energy, our life force, is innocent. It is our expression of the pure and exhilarating desire to be alive. Everything contains this powerful impulse."
—Azra Bertrand and Seren Bertrand[26]

In the same ways that the power of women's bodies has been shut down, the true power of sex has been relegated to some shadowy, far-off corner, only to be met with and understood in the most superficial of ways.

Every single person who exists, has ever existed, and will ever exist comes from the energy of sex. Every human being has spent the beginnings of their existence within the walls of the womb. We've all known the beautiful, dark intimacy of the womb space.

However, as we go out into the world and accumulate experiences, we start shutting down our sexuality and hiding our own natural luster. We cut ourselves off from our vibrant, sensual, and energetic natures. Sex becomes this thing that is separate from who we are.

But how can this really be? Sex is everything. Our sexuality is present in our breath, our cells, and our organs. It is the underpinning of all that we are.

You are a sexual creature who deserves to live life tapped into the source of what you are. You deserve to feel deep ecstatic pleasure, energy, and transformation. You deserve to share this energy with the people you want to share it with.

---

26. Azra Bertrand and Seren Bertrand, *Womb Awakening* (Vermont: Bear & Company, 2017), 23.

For way too many centuries, sex has been used against women. Too many women have been hurt, abused, or killed due to patriarchal structures and mindsets seeking to control our bodies.

When a woman gets older, it's assumed she isn't sexually viable, and society doesn't pay her as much attention as before. However, the older a woman becomes, the more wisdom, confidence, and beauty she starts to inhabit, and the more she steps into her power. We should uphold, honor, and recognize our older women, as they are the ones bringing forth the deeper wisdom and accumulation of experiences.

Our youth-obsessed culture pumps out the narrative that aging is some kind of undesirable abnormality. But it is a natural truth—one that must be embraced and celebrated. As a woman gets older, she has more and more ability to hone and deepen her connection to her sexual energy in a way that is expansive and ever unfolding. No matter what age a woman is, she has the innate ability to tap into her sexual self, to deepen that feeling of being "home" in her own body.

The Sacredness inside You

Whenever you notice a feeling of aliveness inside of you, or a boost of energy within, that is your sexual nature. It's where you come from. It's that madly beautiful spark of electricity that exists inside of you. It's the fire you carry within. It's what makes you who you are. You have a right to own that.

Sexual energy is not something that is only reserved for lovers. It isn't something that must only be expressed behind closed doors in the bedroom, away from curious eyes. Your sexual energy is an ongoing phenomenon that is dancing within you at all times. Sexual energy isn't something that should be solely used for intercourse or intimate encounters.

We've forgotten how sacred we are. We've forgotten that our sexual energy makes up the magical, expansive, and all-encompassing foundation of our lives.

Look at any aspect you struggle with—your relationships, money, negative thoughts, unbalanced emotions. And then consider what your relationship to your sexual energy looks like. How happy are you with the sex you're receiving—or not receiving? How connected do you feel with your sensuality, with your own body? Are you satisfied with the amount and depth of plea-sure you feel in your daily life? Many times, we find that the challenges in our lives can be linked to our feelings and experiences with our sexual energy, and how comfortable we are with our sexuality.

Since our wombs are connected to our sexuality, we can use this sacred part of our bodies to bring in more healing and a deeper connection to and understanding of what sex really means.

What Sexual Energy Really Is

It's as simple as this: sexual energy is life force energy. And life force energy is the vibrancy that you carry within your body at all times. It is the same as source energy, which is the energy that is present in all things. This is the energy that comes from what we know as the Creator, God, or a higher power.

Since we were created from sex, from the merging and fusing of this dynamic life force energy, every cell of our being is laced with sexual vitality.

This sexual vitality is what propels you forward. It's that feeling of bliss when you're completely lost in doing something you love, losing all notion of time and space. It's that deep, intimate connection you feel swelling up in your heart when you go to embrace a loved one whom you're bursting with excitement to see. It's that ecstatic *yes* within when you feel, undeniably, that you are blazing down the right path, at the right time, in just the right way.

Above all, that sexual vitality that exists within you is your presence. It informs how you claim your space in the world. It is the underpinning of all your thoughts, actions, and words. It is your connection to your body, and to other people. It is everything.

And yet, our world has a limited understanding of what sex truly is, and just how much potential and power it holds. The energy of sex has been dis-torted into something dirty, or taboo, or not pure enough.

All of us deserve to receive pleasure, and to know the feeling of also giv-ing it. But it doesn't have to be simply confined to intercourse, or what hap-pens in the bedroom behind closed doors.

When we reserve our sexual expression and our pleasure for our romantic partners, we're setting limits on the potential we can unlock in this lifetime.

Remember, always, that sex is not intercourse; it is an energy that vibrates within you. Take that energy and color your life with it. Make the world your lover. Surrender your body, mind, heart, and spirit to the full experience of each day. Let your senses guide you. Take nothing and no one for granted. Move your body in ways that reflect the rare brilliance of your wild spirit. Judge no one. Send silent blessings to those who hurt you, and don't let your mind get caught up with rehashing the past. Live out your deepest desires and spread love wherever you go.

All of that is the power of sex, of sexual energy. That is the true, unbounded vibrancy that is inherent in our sexual selves.

When you keep a living thing in a dark box forever, you cannot expect that thing to thrive. A living thing contained becomes an unnatural version of itself. Locked in a box, it withers, becomes frayed and twisted. Leave it this way for years, or decades, and it will morph into some hollow version of itself. It will fight to survive by operating in ways that are in sharp contrast to its true nature.

This is what we've done to sex. We've shut it in a dark box and wrung all its magic out. We've stripped it of its essence, dressed it down to some unrecognizable thing.

This is why so many of us have disconnected from our bodies. This is why we've stopped paying attention to our wombs and breasts. This is why we sometimes ignore that wild fluttering in the heart, that sensation that is desperately trying to remind us of what we truly are.

That untamed part of ourselves, that connection to our sexual expression, can feel so far away at times, even though it's right there inside of us.

You can hop on a plane and take dozens of trips to all the world's most exotic and exhilarating places—but none of them will come close to touching the beautiful and thrilling trip that is the inner journey into the soul, the heart, and the womb. No map is required on this trip, and there is no final destination. It is an ongoing unfurling, an ever-expanding quest of inner transformation and waking up to your true power.

That journey within never ends. There isn't a point where you can say, "Okay, been there, done that. Now what?"

Once you start to know yourself in a deeper way, once you begin to open up to your inner space, you start realizing that there is more, always more— that what is available to you is infinite.

Your body is the key here. By owning your sexual expression, you start to own all of yourself. You open up your power in exciting and new ways. More energy and wisdom become accessible, because you start to pay attention to what's present. It's not like they were ever separate from you. This beauty, this magic, has always been there. You just need to take all of it out of the box and into the light, so it can do its thing. So it can support you in unleashing what you are and who you are meant to be.

Ask yourself honestly: Are you living at your fullest potential right now?

Are you cultivating relationships that fill you all the way up to the top and make you dizzy with joy?

Are you speaking your truth?

Are you doing the things that fulfill the wildest desires in your heart, so that when it's time to leave this body, this life, you can think of no regrets?

I hope you are. And if you're not, just place your hands over your womb and breathe. All the way down. Know that you have everything you need inside of you.

Your expression at its fullest is unlike any other on this planet. If you don't use it, then the world will not get to benefit from it. Show up by honoring the calling, the pull, the whisper. Be brave and know that it's safe to step into who you really are.

SHARING ENERGY WITH SEXUAL PARTNERS

Since sexual energy is the foundation for who we are, the parts of our bodies that are used for the act of sex carry a lot of energy. This means that unresolved feelings and struggles can be held in the genital area.

When you allow a sexual partner inside of you, you're taking on all of whom that person is. Sex doesn't merely complete itself after one encounter.

For example, if you are with a partner who has a penis, and you take that penis inside of you, you are also energetically taking on your partner's emotions and experiences. When a partner enters your vagina, that partner brings their emotional world inside of you. That world seeps into the cells of your vagina, and the residue lingers there, long after the sexual encounter.

Since the genitals are places of power and sexuality, information and experiences accumulate in these spaces.

Even if you don't take a lover inside of you, and you are instead being intimate with someone who has a vagina, the energy inside of that yoni will also stay with you.

With sex, you are bringing the energy of someone else's sacred parts to your own sacred parts. Exchanging sexual energy and fluids with another being will, of course, impact your own energy, mood, and vibration. Listen to your inner voice when you're trying to determine whether or not you want to share intimacy with a particular person. Check in with yourself and make sure you feel safe with the person you're connecting with.

During sex, be present to what's occurring inside of you. Do you feel able to bring the most intimate parts of yourself into the act? Do you feel deeply connected, nurtured, safe, and cherished by your partner? Practice the art of listening to the inner wisdom of your body.

Listening to the body's wisdom will help empower you around sex and relationships. Not to mention the fact that it will deepen your connection to yourself and your partner. If you don't have a partner, listening to your inner wisdom can support you in knowing whom you truly want to give your time and energy to.

Another essential thing to understand: a partner does not "make or break" your sexual energy. If you don't currently want a partner in your life, or if you haven't found the right one yet, this should not dictate the ways in which you tap into your sexual energy. Women can be whole and complete without the attention—sexual or otherwise—from a partner. We hold the keys to unlock the heights of pleasure, love, and erotic potential within ourselves.

Our level of fulfillment and pleasure should never be beholden to a partner. It's something we always have inside of us that can be tapped into at any moment. To hinge it all on someone else indicates that we feel we are somehow lacking, or not enough.

But you are enough.

If you ever forget this fact, tune in to your womb, or inside of your breasts, and you will be jolted back into awareness of your true and sacred essence. Do some breast massage, or a yoni steam, or a womb meditation, and acquaint yourself with your power, again and again. Remind yourself of it as much as you need to.

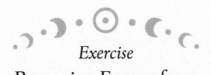

Exercise

Removing Energy from Past Partners out of the Vagina

This exercise is for anyone who wants to cleanse the vagina and release any stuck energies from previous partners. If you were in a relationship with someone who is no longer in your life, and you want to remove any lingering energy that may still be in your vagina, this is the exercise for you. Or if you've had sex with someone that maybe you didn't choose consciously, and you feel you want to remove their energy, this is also a great exercise for you to try.

Keep in mind that it doesn't matter how long it has been since you've been with this partner. It could be someone from a decade ago, or someone you just slept with last night. It also doesn't have to be for one specific person. Perhaps there are multiple partners in your past whom you energetically seek to distance yourself from. You can decide to focus on just one past partner, or multiple past partners.

It also doesn't matter what form of genitalia this former partner has, or whether or not they've physically placed themselves inside of you. Sexual energy clings to the vagina regardless, and so you can do this for any past partner you've had.

Find a comfortable place to lie down on your back. Place both hands over your pelvis. Relax here and just take a few womb breaths.

Set an intention for what you're going to release. You can say this mentally or out loud. What you say exactly is up to you and should be organic to what you feel and want to focus on releasing. For example, you can say, *I release any energy from and attachment to* _____. Feel free to state the name of the person, if you want to be specific. Or you can simply say "my past sexual partners."

Take time to focus on and feel your vagina as you continue to breathe deeply.

Now imagine that your breath is a healing elixir. Take in that healing elixir as you inhale through the nose. Guide that healing elixir all the way down the body to the vagina. As you breathe that healing elixir down, imagine it is healing everything it comes into contact with—your womb, your ovaries, your cervix, your vagina. When you get to the opening of your vagina, hold your breath, and feel the healing elixir caressing the opening of the vagina. When you're ready to exhale, exhale through the mouth, and imagine that the breath is moving out of your body and into the ground beneath you.

Continue this breath at least nine more times.

When you've completed these breaths, focus back on your vagina and notice how it feels.

Speak to your vagina. Say whatever is in your heart. Let your vagina know how cherished it is, and how you promise to be conscious about whom you let inside of it going forward. Let your vagina know how much it matters to you and how grateful you are for all it does.

This is an exercise that can be done whenever you need it. Use it to connect to your vagina and your sexual energy in a deeper way, while also removing all the stuck energies and old dramas you no longer need to carry with you.

DRAWING CONSCIOUS LOVING PARTNERSHIPS TO YOU

Cherish your womb. Become more loving and aware of your body. When you do this, you heal. You create more joyful, high-vibrating feelings within. Your thoughts become laced with positive and empowering tones.

When you start opening up to the magic of what you are, you become irresistible. You begin to attract other people, experiences, and situations that are in alignment with the positive energy you're cultivating inside of yourself.

If you're looking for a conscious, loving partnership, tune in to your womb space. Place your hands over your vulva (or pelvic area) and silently bless it each day. Vow to care for it, and ask it to support you in staying conscious of the lovers you allow inside of you.

If you already are in a loving partnership, you can work with your womb to help you continue reaching new heights of divine love and awareness. Fill your womb up with positive thoughts and loving energies simply by imagining them inside of your womb. The more positivity and love you can shine down into your womb, the more healing and pleasure you start to open up within yourself. Send blessings to your vagina as well, and give gratitude for all your vagina has experienced during your lifetime.

Your body is a gift, and a way of knowing your power as a woman on this planet. Praise every inch of your physical being. Don't get fixated on what you deem imperfect or not good enough. All of that is just our culture's shallow definitions of beauty interfering with your mind. Slice away your attachment to what society thinks, and claim ownership over your body and sexuality.

Past Sexual Abuse and Violence

Recently, the World Health Organization shared that almost one in every three women, during their lifetime, is subjected to physical or sexual violence from a partner, or sexual violence from a non-partner.[27]

One in three women.

Violence against women is something that happens every day in every country across our world, yet we've become numb to it. Black women disproportionately experience more violence in their homes and communities. Data shows that, in their lifetime, four out of ten Black women experience physical violence from an intimate partner.[28]

Women and girls became especially more vulnerable after the start of the COVID-19 pandemic, due to lockdowns and the inability to normally access vital services. This is an emergency of mass proportions, one that our world is not really making a priority to deal with.

If you've had past experiences of physical or sexual violence, if you've ever had to endure sexual abuse or rape, know that there are countless amazing and strong women, like yourself, who are also struggling with similar experiences. Women have endured massive amounts of pain and cruelty for way too long. We've been expected to carry so many burdens. But the thing is, our spirits are strong. And even though our relationships to our bodies and our sexual energy might have been impacted by past negative experiences, they don't define who we are. We get to define who we are. We get to heal, we get to thrive, we get to fulfill our biggest and boldest desires. And we get to do all of this on our own terms.

27. "Devastatingly pervasive: 1 in 3 women globally experience violence,"World Health Organization, March 9, 2021, https://www.who.int/news/item/09-03-2021-devastatingly-pervasive-1-in-3-women-globally-experience-violence.

28. Susan Green, "Violence Against Black Women—Many Types, Far-reaching Effects," Institute for Women's Policy Research, July 13, 2017, https://iwpr.org/iwpr-issues/race-ethnicity-gender-and-economy/violence-against-black-women-many-types-far-reaching-effects/.

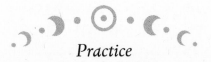

Practice

Cutting Ties from Past Sexual Violence, Abuse, or Rape

This practice involves taking a bath and is for healing from past sexual violence, abuse, or rape. It isn't necessary to relive any past experiences during this healing bath. Just connect with your body and trust that it knows exactly what it needs to release at this time.

Here's what you'll need for this healing experience:

- Bathtub
- Candles and lighter
- Rose petals (optional)
- Essential oil (optional)
- Clear quartz crystal (optional)

Light some candles and draw a hot bath for yourself.

If you have any rose petals, place these in the bath now. If you want to put a drop or two of an essential oil, like lavender, you can do that as well. Place any quartz crystals you have into the bath with you also. These are only optional, so if you don't have any of these readily available, you don't need to add them to your bath. It will not lessen this practice in any way. The important thing here is that you have access to a bath.

Once everything is ready, you can go ahead and get into the bath. Relax here and just breathe. As you sit in the bath, go through these steps...

Set an intention. You can say something like, *My vagina and womb release all* _____. Or, *My pelvic area releases all* _____. And then fill in the blank with whatever you choose.

Allow yourself to focus on your womb and vagina. Imagine that the water is cleansing your womb and vagina and ridding them of any stuck emotions, feelings, or energies. Feel all those negative past energies and experiences being absorbed and cleansed by the water.

At the end of the bath, place your left hand over your womb and your right hand over your vagina. Breathe here and silently (or quietly) state your intention from earlier, but this time, state it as something that has just happened. Here's an example: *My womb and vagina have released* _____.

By using *have released*, you're stating the intention as if it's something that has just occurred, as opposed to stating it as something in the present tense, or something that's in the process of happening.

After this, you can sit in the bath for a bit longer if you like, or you can come out.

This practice can be done as often as you like. Water's transformational nature has the ability to heal, cleanse, and purify. Adding any oils, rose petals, or crystals into the mix will help the purification along, but as I mentioned, this is not necessary if you don't have access to any of those items.

NOT HAVING SEX

During our lives, we'll go through periods in which we're not having a whole lot of sex, or any at all, in some cases. Whether it's because we're currently not in a relationship, or we're in a relationship in which sex has waned, or we simply don't have the energy or interest in it, there's no reason to feel as if you're lacking somehow.

We can use our sexual energy in so many different ways. Remember, sex isn't just about having intercourse with another human being. It was never meant to be confined into one very specific box. Our sexual energy is our life force energy, and it is tied to everything we do, think, speak, and create.

*It is our birthright to cultivate and express
our sexual energy out in the world, and
not just with romantic partners.*

Don't shut down that part of yourself just because you're not having physical sex in your life at the moment. If you shut down that part of yourself, you risk cutting out your natural vibrancy, energy, and sensuality. All this is vital to who you are. It's that inherent spark you carry within. Don't dull this down or lose touch with it just because you aren't having intercourse.

Fuel your life with sexual vitality. Open up your senses. Allow yourself to feel every feeling and emotion. Become wildly aware of your body, and listen to those inner whispers within. Do a daily breast massage, engage in self-touch, and send loving thoughts to your womb. All these things will enhance your sexual energy and tap you into a deeper current of life.

When you do all these things, you start to engage with your senses, breath, and body in a different way. This will allow a natural vibration to well up within you. At first, it might be so subtle that you won't notice it. But as you start paying more attention to your body, you will naturally start to notice all the small sensations you might not have recognized before.

Allow yourself to become enamored by the subtle shifts within you. See them fully and completely for what they are, and don't take them for granted as they come. Every flutter in your heart, or rush of warmth in your belly, or tightening in your calves is telling you something.

*Every feeling within you is a calling to
come back to yourself.*

You hold immense sexual electricity within. This belongs to no one else but you. You can use it to do what you please.

Once you start to notice this sexual energy, this vibration, this wild current running through you, take it and transmute it. Stay tapped into the center of it and use it to fuel all your projects and pursuits.

In your relationships, use this energy, this electricity, to have conversations, to cultivate closeness, and to forge new territory with your loved ones. When you share your sexual energy with everyone—and not just a romantic partner—your relationships start to take on a more exciting texture. Work this vitality in to all your relationships and watch your bonds and connections between loved ones in your life blossom.

This sexual vitality can also be used to feed your creative projects, your work, and any action you take with an effusive kind of potency. Bringing your sexual energy into your pursuits and experiences means you're taking the definition of sex out of the box.

Sex is deep integration with all of life, where the entire world is your lover. Where ecstatic bliss is inherent in every moment. Where you see and know yourself in a more vibrant way, and where you honor the sacred reality that exists inside of you.

When you let your sexual energy move out to the world around you, the heart at the center of your life starts to beat at a different pace. You start to flow, to relax and release at greater levels than ever before. You begin to live your fullest life. Inner peace, joy, beauty, and pleasure become your natural state.

So how do you do this? How do you amplify your sexual energy and bring it out into the world around you?

The answer is through your womb and your breasts. These parts of yourself are gateways into the center of your sexual energy. This energy permeates every cell in your being, but it is even more concentrated in your womb and your breasts. To unfurl the energies in these places, you've got to employ the healing and rejuvenating powers of self-care. Caring for your breasts and your womb automatically lets your body know you are aware of the sacred power it holds. It's an acknowledgment of your deep divine nature. You start to experience your body as a temple, and when you do this, it sets off a chain reaction that ignites all your sexual energy and unspools the fullest potential of your ability to love yourself.

To care for your breasts, use some of the practices that have been shared in this book. Yoni steaming, breast massage, deep breathing, and womb meditations are all ways to unlock the fullest expression of your sexual energy.

When you unlock your sexual energy, you don't have to focus on being starved for sex, or feeling sexually inadequate, or feeling guilty or ashamed of your body. You don't have to feel lacking of any touch. You don't have to pine or yearn for another to unlock the magic that you are. *Because you've already unlocked it.*

Once you unlock it, it's hard to look back. When your sexual power is unleashed, a new kind of life starts to bubble up inside of you.

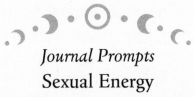

Journal Prompts
Sexual Energy

Grab your Womb Journal or some paper and prepare to write about and reflect on your sexual energy.

Drink a glass of water before you start writing. This will help put you in a flow state with your writing and will also activate the energy in the womb. Remember, water is the element of the womb space, and it is incredibly healing and necessary for sustaining our feminine systems and bodies.

Before you start, set an intention to allow your heart and your womb to fuel your writing. Feel the energies of the womb move up into the heart, and from there, allow the intermingled energies of heart and womb to pour through your arms, into your hands, and out onto the paper.

Write your responses to the following questions:

- What does my current relationship to my sexual energy look like?
- Am I only reserving my sexual energy for sex, or do I use it in other aspects of my life? If I do use my sexual energy in other aspects of my life, how and where exactly am I using it?

- What, if anything, is holding me back from expressing my sexual energy?
- What would my daily life look like if I allowed the full height of my sexual energy to be expressed?

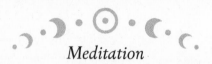

Meditation

Freeing Your Sexual Energy

This is a great meditation for bringing your sexual energy up to the surface.

Lie down on your back. Place a pillow under your knees for comfort, if you need to. Allow your arms to extend at your sides and your palms to open up, facing the sky.

Start to take deep womb breaths.

Now, as you continue to breathe deeply through the nose, imagine that a nice, warm sun is shining down on your vagina. Feel the warmth penetrating every part of your vagina, relaxing it and enveloping it in its glow. Allow your vagina to completely melt and relax as this warmth spreads across it. Do this for a few minutes, or longer, if you like the feeling and want to stay with it.

Now, on your next inhale, send that breath through the nose and all the way down into your vagina, right into the center of that warmth.

Hold your breath here for a few seconds as you focus in on the vagina, on all that warmth radiating within it.

And when you're ready, start to exhale out the nose and imagine that the warmth from your vagina is spreading out in all directions, across your entire body. Feel that warmth, that vibrancy, as it envelops your whole being.

Do this breath for five to ten minutes.

Try not to rush this breath. Go slowly, and allow yourself to stay present to all the warmth and sensation moving through you.

When you've completed this meditation, stay there on your back and just feel into your body. Notice all the newness that has been awakened within you. If you feel any sensation or vibration in your body, pay attention to it. Give it your full awareness and breathe into it. Honor each ripple within you, no matter how tiny and insignificant it might seem. Let each sensation wrap itself around your entire being. This is your sexual energy, your own unique vibration. Amplify it with your focus and attention.

Channeling Your Sexual Energy

Once you've awakened your sexual energy, you've got to take it out into your daily life. Again, reserving it for sexual encounters means you're inhibiting a major part of who you are from being seen by the rest of the world. Taking your sexual energy out into the world doesn't mean you're physically attempting to make love to everyone you see. Instead, it means you approach life in a state of perpetual joy, surrender, and adventure. It means you are energetically creating love everywhere you step. Sexual energy is that spark of aliveness that exists inside of you, and instead of inhibiting it, you are choosing to light the world up with it.

At first, it might appear tricky to fully understand what it means to channel your sexual energy and to put it into everything you do. But once you start doing it, it becomes something so natural that you cannot help but show up as your truest, fullest self.

The easiest way to start using your sexual energy in your life is to first do a practice to align to your sexual energy. You can do the meditation for freeing your sexual energy, or you can even do a breast meditation or massage. You can even shake your body out, or just turn on some music and dance.

Movement stirs sexual energy awake.

Movement brings vitality into your cells and puts them in motion. If you can dance every morning, it will open your sexual energy and bring your body into a receptive and energized state. That buzz of energy we feel humming within after dancing is that sexual energy we want to grab hold of and align to. Since practices and meditations involving our breasts and our wombs contain greater amounts of this energy, we can work with them to go deeper and more precisely target our sexual vitality within. But there's nothing like dancing or shaking for a few minutes to also start bringing that sexual energy to the surface.

Once you feel that energy thrumming through your body, don't make the mistake of losing connection to it and going about your day. After you dance, meditate, or massage yourself, you've got to take the time to pause, to be still, and to breathe into the energy. This is an important way to start integrating the energy and taking it out into the world with you.

Too often, we do the yoga practice, or the meditation practice, and then we go about our normal days, leaving this energy behind. We don't know how to integrate it and how to use it moment to moment. We lose connection to it, and we don't merge the practice into our daily lives.

It's time to stop compartmentalizing practices that nurture, soothe, and heal. Let your body be the bridge that actualizes these practices out into the world.

After you've made time for stillness to connect with the sexual energy you've stirred up within you, go about your day, and continue to stay aligned to that vibration within. Attempt to stay present and aware. Don't let your thoughts bog you down and pull you away from that inner connection.

When you have a conversation with someone, work on a project, sit at your computer, clean your house, or whatever else you do, let that vitality within you guide your actions, your motions, and your words. Staying present and plugged in to this energy might take a few tries, but be gentle with yourself and keep making a commitment to align to your sexual power.

Once you get the hang of it, and you're able to stay plugged in, you might notice that the feeling of sexual energy starts to take on a certain kind of depth. You might also notice that it starts to just naturally be present for you, without you having to engage in any methods of movement or visualization to bring it to the surface. Reaching this point will naturally keep your energy awake, which means you don't have to worry about doing a practice or exercise to incite this energy before you work with it. You can still make time for practices, but it doesn't have to be a daily thing, if you don't have the time.

When I started working with and channeling my sexual energy, I felt as if I was in the midst of some wild and unchartered exploration. I began the practices with no clue as to what I was doing really. I just had a desire to know myself in a deeper way. Just by breathing and focusing on my breasts, I unleashed this current of energy within that both startled and fascinated me. I had never experienced my sexual energy in this way before. It felt as if it had no boundaries.

After awakening that energy, I went deeper into my explorations. Years later, I continue to feel my sexual energy moving full-force through my body. It's like a vibration of pleasure, bliss, and perpetual peace beating through me at all times. I wouldn't trade this feeling for any other feeling in the world.

Although the energy is awake within me, I still carve out time to do practices. Keeping a consistent practice helps you stay present and aligned to your body and sexual energy. Find the path that works for you, and go for it.

PROTECTING YOUR SEXUAL ENERGY

Your sexual energy is sacred. Cultivating it can feel like a thrilling journey. You start to know and understand yourself and your abilities in a whole new way. It becomes crystal clear to you just how limitless you truly are.

At the same time, protecting your sexual energy is an absolute must. Send your sexual energy out to projects, people, and experiences that excite and embolden you. Channel it in ways that make you feel loved and cherished. Protect it from people and experiences that aren't in your highest good and do nothing to nurture your spirit and heart.

It might be difficult, in the beginning, to discern where to put your energy, and where not to put it. The thing about being aligned to your sexual energy is that it also awakens your feminine strengths. Intuition is one of those strengths. Our intuition encompasses our ability to make decisions and to know what the right path is. Sexual energy opens up the body and wakes up this innate intelligence within it.

You know how you meet somebody for the first time, and there's this feeling inside of you that this is a person you'd really love to get to know? Or maybe you get presented with a big opportunity at work, and you're tempted to grab it, but then there's this voice inside that tells you it wouldn't be for you, that you'd be sacrificing way too much time and energy for it?

All of that is the voice of your intuition. Some of us can't hear it all the time. And for some of us, even if we do hear it, we don't always listen to it. We might falter or hesitate to heed our inner calling, because we worry that if we don't make decisions from a logical place, we'll be ruining our lives. But intuition doesn't ruin life, it enhances it.

Intuition is part of our feminine gifts, and we can use it to navigate our lives in a meaningful way.

Your intuition will support you in protecting your sexual energy. Listen to that voice within, and don't push it aside. It will communicate directly to you and let you know where you should be putting your energy. Tune in to your body, and you will hear your intuition speak to you.

Let's say you meet a potential romantic partner. This partner may be beautiful and amazing on the outside, but when you go to talk to them, you might feel this sensation deep in your body, pulling you in the opposite direction, away from this person. That's your intuition. Despite the attraction, your intuition simply knows this is not a person you want to go any deeper with. The same kinds of examples can be used for meeting new friends, making career choices, or any number of other decisions that consume us each day.

Protecting your sexual energy means honoring your intuition. Don't give your energy to people and things that don't elevate you. Give your energy to people and things that light you up and bring out the best in you.

And remember, your sexual energy doesn't just pertain to sex or romantic partnerships. Sexual energy is your own innate vitality, and when you share it, you are sharing a sacred part of yourself. Pour this energy into the people and things you love, and watch your life become pure magic.

CHAPTER 12 TAKEAWAYS

- Sexual energy shouldn't be reserved for the bedroom. It should be taken out into the world and used to infuse our encounters, experiences, projects, and relationships.
- Our genitals carry energy and information from our past sexual or romantic partners.
- It's essential to work on removing any accumulated energies from past lovers and experiences so that we can more deeply experience ourselves and our sexual energy.
- Amplify your sexual energy and channel it out into your daily life. Make time for practices like breast massage, yoni steaming, and womb meditations.
- Always work to protect your sexual energy. It's a sacred part of who you are.

Chapter 13

A FULFILLING
SEX LIFE

"Sex is about as close to ourselves as we can get; it reaches, touches, and changes every cell of our bodies."
       —Diana Richardson[29]

Since we explored sexual energy in the last chapter, you have an understanding of how powerful that vitality within can be; and how, when we use it toward means that aren't just hinged on sex, the potential for transformation is tremendous.

Taking that vitality, that inner sexual energy, and bringing it into our sexual encounters brings the act of sex to a whole other level. Being in tune with your own orgasmic energy and fueling that toward lovemaking with a partner you care deeply about becomes an intoxicating, out-of-this-world experience.

If we don't align to our own sensuality, we not only feel disconnected from our partners during sex, but we are also disconnected from ourselves. You can't find satisfaction this way. You've got to first harness and plug into your own deep well of pleasure within. Only then can you truly connect with your partner.

You know that thing they say about people who are unable to love themselves? If you don't love yourself, how can you ever really give and express love

---

29. Diana Richardson, *Tantric Orgasm for Women* (Vermont: Destiny Books, 2004), 4.

to someone else? You can try, and maybe even succeed at it for some time. But you will hit a wall. You cannot ever give something you don't possess within.

Deep sexual fulfillment must always start with the self. Understand how to cultivate and circulate your sexual energy. Know where and how you like to be touched. Let that warmth and vitality flood across the womb and breasts. Understand the sexual language within your own body. Open your senses in ways that elevate your sexual awareness.

Once you've done all that, you can start to bring your partner into the mix and begin the journey of deepening and enhancing your sex life. And if you don't have a partner, that's fine, too; finding that orgasmic pleasure within yourself will fulfill you in ways you probably never thought were possible.

Many of us didn't grow up ever hearing anything remotely like this. To know that we are in charge of our own sexual pleasure puts us in an empowering position.

The messages we've picked up about sex during our lifetimes have been tainted with misinformation and misogynist preferences. Marinating in these toxic ideas has led us to disconnect from our bodies, our sexual vitality, and our truest selves.

But we have a chance to flip that script. To change things up for the better. To see to it that we receive the kind of sexual pleasure and satisfaction we deserve.

Women are queens of sensuality, beauty, and ecstasy. Our wombs have never forgotten what we truly are. These energies are innate qualities that always exist within us, longing to be known and expressed. We just need to come home to the erotic adventure that lives and breathes inside of us.

There is no rigid and calculated map when it comes to traversing the inner world of the body. Since this is feminine terrain, the quest is a multilayered one. It has no straight, hard lines to obediently walk and follow. The feminine journey is a cyclical and multifaceted experience. It has no final destination. It is a wild cycling of inner pleasure, mysticism, and expansiveness.

THE TYPICAL WAY WE DO ORGASMS

During sex, a whole lot of tension, buildup, and excitement are crammed toward achieving one main purpose—an orgasm. Reaching orgasm is a kind of obsession that many of us fixate on, to the exclusion of all the subtle energies and sensations inside our bodies.

When we focus on the end result of orgasm, we lose the ability to truly connect with ourselves and our partners. This kind of one-track focus on the desired end result also keeps us from experiencing longer, more satisfying orgasms.

Focusing on creating sensation in the genital area actually restricts us from experiencing deep, expansive pleasure. All it does is create tension in the body, which limits our sexual energy from being expansive and circulating inside of us. Since sexual energy is your life force energy, and the energy by which you can feel your natural sense of aliveness, it only makes sense that you would allow this energy to move through your entire body during the act of sex.

By applying limits to sexual energy, by focusing solely on your vagina or genital area, you are restricting it. You're placing it in a very small box, yet at the same time expecting to feel overwhelmed with ecstasy. But that's not gonna happen. Not when your sexual energy is contained and confined to one area. Not when the act of sex is a game of tension, buildup, and release.

When we think about hot sex, we tend to think about a fast and hard approach. If you have a vagina and your preference is to take a man inside of you, he might be very mechanical in the way he makes love to you—that rapid in-and-out motion, that feeling of heat and tension. You can feel pleasure this way, but it will skate on the surface of what is possible. So many of us are used to having sex in this way that we don't question it.

Once excitement builds its way to a quick genital orgasm and is released, your sexual vitality is moved out of you. It's not free to circulate and move through the body, which can often leave us with a hollow feeling after the act. That feeling of something not quite being right.

Continuing to approach sex this way will eventually turn us off completely. Some of us might already be completely turned off, might have no desire for sex at all. Having a whole lot of unfulfilling sex can do that to you. If you identify with that feeling of numbness and disinterest when it comes to sex, know that this doesn't have to be your reality forever.

*A woman needs nourishing sex that goes
beyond the confines of her body and reaches out
to encompass her heart and soul.*

Women need to be cherished, nurtured, and appreciated. When sex becomes tangled up in expectations, a woman can lose her ability to feel herself and to expand her sexual energy.

The problem is, sex has yet to be widely embraced as a holistic way of connecting to the self, to a partner, and, by extension, to the entire universe. It's not widely thought of as a source of empowerment, as a way of building and sustaining your vitality, as a way of honoring and loving the deepest parts of yourself.

But it is all of this, and so much more.

*Sex is a way of knowing the self and the body at
a deeper level. It's a way of merging with not only
your partner, but the universe as a whole.*

Sex is an adventure, and an opportunity to express the fullest self. It's a way of integrating body, mind, spirit, and heart. And it's a healthy form of expression that promotes well-being, joy, balance, and flow in one's life.

This is a sacred, tantric way of approaching sex. Tantra is actually a deep spiritual practice of meditation that has been around for thousands of years. It was first created in India and has spread to other parts of the world. A tantric practice is based upon working with your energy centers, your breath, and your body to awaken life force energy within. And since that life force energy is, at its essence, sexual energy, the principles of tantra have been taken and incorporated into the act of sex.

Does applying some tantric practices to your sex life mean you are taking on a new religion of some kind? It doesn't, as tantra is not a religion. The principles of tantra are based in coming home to yourself, in waking up to the power of your own body. It is a sacred way of understanding yourself and your sexuality, of following the call of that inner voice within.

Oftentimes, in our world, we try to label things so that they fit neatly into boxes. But our sexuality is anything but neat, and it certainly doesn't belong in a box. There's a natural vibration, a wild kind of current that is always running through you; one that defies definition. This unspooling and activating of your sexual energy is a deeply personal inward journey that does not conform to a logical, linear structure. It breaks free of structure and operates by following the innate cyclical integrity of your feminine nature.

Since sexual energy is not dependent upon whether or not you're having sex, you can always work with it and circulate it on your own. For those of us who don't have a partner or don't want to have a partner at this time, I highly recommend you stay connected to your sexual energy and continue to build it and experience it. You can use the exercises I share in the chapter on sexual energy. You can also use the exercises in the following section of this chapter to learn more deeply how to tune in to, amplify, and circulate your sexual energy.

For those of you who want to use sexual energy with a current or future partner as a way of deepening your sex life, the exercises in this chapter will support you in doing that. Follow the solo practices first, and then take what you've learned into your bedroom—or wherever your preferable location for sex may be!

GOING SOLO

Before you can cultivate a sex life that makes you feel like the smoking hot goddess you are, you must start within. Our partners are an important half of the equation for sure. But before you venture on this path together, you've got to be able to relax into your own sexual energy and start to work with it. Learning how to circulate your sexual energy is an essential way to stay aware and in tune with your inner being.

Practice
Unlock the Energy in Your Breasts

The source of your sexual energy is located in your breasts. You can liberate that energy with some breast massage. If you don't have breasts, you can still do this exercise and get the benefits of the practice. Direct your attention to the inside of your chest area. Again, try not to focus on the outside, over the skin of the chest, but guide that energy toward the inner world of your chest. You don't need physical breasts to tap this rich and wild energy. It's contained within your heart space and carries tremendous power.

If you do have breasts, cup them in the palms of your hands and shake them out to clear stagnant energies. As you do this, meditate on your breasts; focus on feeling them and sensing them on the inside of your body, as opposed to the outside.

A high amount of sensation and vibration can be felt within the breasts, so the more time you devote to them, the more you'll start to sense those subtle energies moving within. In the beginning, you might notice very little. But I promise you, if you stick with it, you'll unearth a wave of orgasmic pleasure inside of you. Once you align to it, you'll think you've hit your limit. But it will just continue to expand and grow. It's just like doing exercise. We keep our bodies fit by consistently showing up to work out and take care of ourselves. By focusing your attention on your breasts, you're working to expand and cultivate your sexual energy, which is the foundation for your whole being.

THE SENSATION

Once you start to feel that sense of vibration in the breasts, it's time to start moving and circulating it through the body. Doing so is what will bring you into deeper sexual bliss. When you circulate your sexual energy through the body, orgasm is no longer contained. It spreads out to envelop every cell.

To begin circulating your sexual energy, you must first funnel all your focus into your breasts. Once you feel any hint of sensation or vibration, you want to sharpen your focus even more. Wrap your attention around that sensation in your breasts.

If you're not exactly sure what to look out for, here are some examples: a tingling, a warmth, a vibration, a fluttering, a spreading. You want to really tune everything else out so you can be aware of that sensation.

When doing this, you might be a little uncertain. As you begin the journey of developing awareness of your body, you might not notice all the subtle sensations swirling inside of you. But continue to sit in stillness and stay present. Let yourself release all pressure to find or discover anything. There's no set destination in this journey. Let each moment you're sitting in be *the* moment. Let the journey be the focal point of your fascination. Lose yourself in the now. If you are seeking sensation, it might be tough to uncover. Instead, revel in the simple beauty of the moment you're sitting in. Allow each moment to unfold as it needs to. Let the sensation find you when it's ready.

Starting to Move the Energy

Once the sensation has found you, just breathe.

Imagine you are sitting in the center of this sensation. Every part of you is focused so intently on the sensation that your entire being is becoming it. Let the sensation swallow you up, so that there is nothing else that matters in this very moment. To keep yourself anchored in the sensation, start to breathe deeply into it. Feel yourself merge with this sensation as you devote your full attention to it. Let yourself become one with it. Let that focus be a kind of meditation that carries you away into the fullness of the moment.

At this point, you might start to notice the sensation growing larger and starting to expand beyond one point and out to the body. If you don't notice this yet, try to direct the energy with your breath and intention. Take a deep inhale through the nose, and guide that inhale down into the center of the sensation. Once it's there, hold it, as if trying to gather or pool the energy present there. When you exhale, imagine the energy is spreading out from that sensation to the entire body around it. Instead of going into any one single direction, imagine the energy is leaking from all directions out across your body. Feel the sensation spread out around to your entire being.

Continue this breath to keep moving the energy through your body.

Just by using your intention, you allow yourself to develop a deeper awareness of your sexual energy.

Be sure to take both your inhale and exhale slowly, so that you can really feel the energy. Going too fast might disconnect you from the present moment and from your body. Keep it slow, and stay present to the process.

Starting to Circulate the Energy

Now it's time to start circulating that energy through the body.

The spine is your main energy pathway in the body. Since it's connected to our chakra points—our major energy centers in the body—it offers a great route for moving and distributing energy. And since the spine is rooted down into the pelvis—which holds so much of our sexual power—it's an ideal path to circulate energy through.

After you've pinpointed the sensation in your heart and have started to move the energy, let go of that focus for a moment. Instead, bring your attention into your cervix, which is located just past your vaginal canal. It is the lowest portion of the womb. According to the chakra system, this part is known to carry our root energy. Our root energy is tied up in our sense of stability, security, home, and money. Sexual energy is also contained in the root area and can be connected to just by focusing on the cervix, as well as on the vaginal muscles.

Take some womb breaths as you keep your attention on the cervix and the vaginal muscles.

Now, to gather the energy, take an inhale and clench the muscles of your cervix and vagina, pulling them in an upward motion. Exhale and unclench the muscle. Try this a few times and notice how your body feels as you do this. It might take some getting used to. If it feels awkward, you can start out by doing a light clench. As you get more accustomed to this practice, you can begin to deepen your clench, if you like.

After you've tried this clench a few times, you're ready to start circulating it through the body. This time, when you inhale and clench the cervix, imagine you're pulling sexual energy from the cervix, all the way up the spine, and to the top of the head. Then, as you exhale, you can unclench the muscles as you imagine you're guiding that energy down the front of the body and back into the cervix. Keep repeating this breath for at least five to ten minutes.

Keep both your inhale and exhale through the nose. Any time you get distracted, just keep coming back to the breath and the body. As you direct the energy upward, be mindful of each part of the spine it touches on its way to the top of the head.

You might find this tricky at first. If it's challenging to do the clenching or you have difficulty concentrating on circulating the energy, take it real slow. Maybe try it for only a minute, and then the next time you can build your way to two minutes.

THAT'S ALL IT TAKES

Once you've tried all these solo steps, you're ready to integrate some of this energy and wisdom into your sex life. That is, only if you want to! The solo practices work wonders in and of themselves and can be used to keep our connection to this tantalizing sexual life force energy within us going strong.

After you've finished these practices, try to find ways to bring all the energy you've accumulated out into your life. Take a moment to sit with the sensations that have been stirred up by the practices, and just breathe into them. Surrender and align to them. Then go about your day, but don't disconnect from all the vitality bursting inside of you. Stay plugged in to it throughout the day by being conscious of your body and your breathing.

Doing this will help you integrate these energies into your life so that you're able to speak, think, act, and express from this wildly rich universe pulsing within you. It will color all your encounters and experiences with a special kind of glow.

WITH A PARTNER, DURING SEX

After working with the solo practices, you can use these practices to deepen and enhance your lovemaking with a partner.

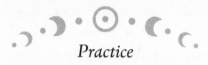

Practice

Be in Your Breasts

With so much attention placed on the vagina during sex, the opportunity to feel a deeper, more intoxicating orgasm is consistently missed. Relegating sexual energy to that one specific genital area limits the amount of pleasure and sensation and takes us out of our bodies.

During sex, we want to be in our bodies. Especially in our breasts, which are the gateway toward feeling true sexual ecstasy in the body. Many have assumed that the clitoris is the way to increase orgasm and sensation, but our feminine bodies don't naturally hold our sexual energy potential in this place. Pay too much attention to the clitoris, and, again, you will limit the amount of sexual energy and push the potential of deep orgasm farther away.

Redirect your attention away from your vagina (for now) and find your home inside your breasts. It's just like what you did during the solo practice, only now, you're bringing it into the act of sex.

As soon as the sexual encounter starts, drop your mind down into your breasts, feeling into both at the same time. This doesn't mean you're going to be out to lunch during sex with your partner. It doesn't mean you won't be present to what's happening in the moment. It means you'll be more available to the moment.

Being present in your own body allows you to be fully present to the moment. When you're in full awareness of your own body, that awareness extends out to everything and everyone around you. Your connection to your inner world amplifies your connection to your outer world. Everything comes into focus. And so, by simply being in your breasts, you bring a state of deep, wild presence to your partner and to the act of lovemaking.

Bring this awareness to your sex life, and it will take on new dimensions and layers. It will excite and delight you in ways that surpass what even the imagination can hold.

Your breasts are the doorway. Use them. Become so present inside of them that you forget any sense of self-consciousness, doubt, or fear. Become so present inside of your breasts that all the other parts of you disappear.

Breathe also. Nice and deep, and through the nose. Your breath will keep you connected to your breasts and your body.

Bringing the breasts into the equation, letting them be the focus of sex, changes everything. It is an untangling and a liberation of your deepest feminine pleasure.

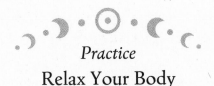

Practice
Relax Your Body

Somehow, conventional sex has mostly become a tight, pounding, mechanical affair. Keeping our eyes on the prize—the highly sought-after orgasm—pulls us out of our bodies and into our heads. It puts us in a state of building tension in the body. It pulls our attention away from all parts of the body just so we can focus on the genital area. But that's not where all the action is. A great deal of our sexual energy is contained in the breasts, and so, we miss out on liberating all of it if our attention goes solely to the vagina.

Instead of creating tension in your body in an effort to achieve that one result, just relax. Let your body be loose. Let it melt into the surface beneath you. When the body is relaxed, more pleasure and energy can flow through it. If the body is tight and tense, all that energy has no way of moving through the body.

Imagine you have a straw. You're about to use it to take a sip of a smoothie you've been dying to drink. Now, imagine that right before you get a chance to have a sip, you take both of your hands and tighten them into two fists around the straw. This would obstruct the straw. So, when you try to drink your smoothie, you might get very little coming through the straw, or even nothing at all. Which is why no one does this. It makes zero sense.

And yet we do this every time we're tensing up our bodies to illicit orgasm. We do this every time we set expectations and focus on our genital areas as a way of strictly fulfilling those expectations. We restrict our own innate orgasmic flow and the potential for truly expanding our pleasure.

At first, it might seem strange to relax your body during sex. You might feel as if you're being lazy and not putting in all the "hard work." But as you relax, you'll start to feel something happening inside of your body. An unrestricted wave of orgasm. A tingling sensation that spreads throughout not only your body, but your whole being.

While in the act of sex, you might need to scan your body at first to determine whether or not you're holding tension anywhere. We can get so accustomed to holding tension in our bodies that we don't even notice we're doing it. Once you start becoming more conscious of relaxing during sex, you'll begin to uncover all the tight parts of your body. Along with your genital area, you might find you hold tension in your jaw, or your neck, or your thighs. As you find these tension points, consciously make an effort to release and relax them.

Let your body soften and surrender.

The more you relax, the more sensation and orgasm you will feel.

Practice

Slow Down

Naturally, as you relax during sex, you'll also start to slow down. Conventional sex can be a very quick process, one that doesn't give women the ample time needed to be present in our bodies.

How many of us reading right now have faked an orgasm at least once? Women want to please their partners, and sometimes, if that means letting them believe we've "come," when in fact we haven't, we'll fake it. Since the motions of conventional sex go against the natural, innate rhythms of our feminine bodies, this can stir up feelings of inadequacy within us.

But, as women, the last thing we are is inadequate. We must stop struggling to keep up with systems that go against our feminine nature. When something doesn't feel good inside the body, that's our cue to abandon whatever it is that incited that feeling—and *move on*.

Women need time to fully immerse themselves in the act. We need time to allow ourselves to steep in the ocean of pleasure and orgasm. When we have sex with someone, we want to be transported to the deepest states of pleasure. But conventional sex puts pleasure in a very tiny box. It makes the whole act of sex hurried, tense, and full of impossible expectations. I say "impossible," because there's no way you can reach the full heights of pleasure by approaching sex in the same superficial ways.

When we slow everything down, this increases the amount of sensation we're able to feel. It puts us more in the moment and keeps us present to the breath and to the body. Why rush in the first place? When orgasm is full and unrestricted—the way it's meant to be—you want it to last.

When you rush, the result is a quick genital orgasm that is composed of built-up tension that is then pushed out of the body in a single unspectacular release. But doing the opposite—relaxing, taking your time, and allowing orgasm to fill up every cell in your body—becomes an awe-inspiring experience that words could never do justice expressing.

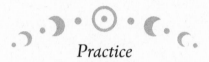

Practice

Be Conscious of Your Breathing

Breathing fully and deeply keeps us present. During sex, let your breath provide the foundation of your awareness and your pleasure. Breathe into your womb space. Be mindful of when you might be holding your breath. If you do find you're holding your breath, that might mean you're holding on to some unnecessary tightness in your body. Restricting the breath is just another way of creating more tension inside you. And more tension means less orgasmic flow.

The more aware you are of your breath, the more in tune you'll be with your body and the present moment.

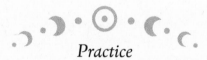

Practice

The Vagina Is Not the Focal Point

By now, you know your vagina shouldn't be the focal point when it comes to your pleasure. Start with your breasts and allow that sexual energy to rise within you. Once it begins in the breasts, it starts to move to encompass other parts of your body, the vagina included. You might start to realize your vagina is becoming wet simply by giving your attention to your breasts.

Remember, the breasts are the gateway. Use the gateway to usher in orgasmic flow, and that flow will start to naturally move through the body.

Once that sexual energy is moving and activated within your body, you can let your focus expand to contain other areas of pleasure inside of you. There isn't a set playbook for this. Try not to be rigid in thinking that since the breasts are the gateway, you have to stay locked into them at all times. Go with the moment. In the beginning, it's good to recognize and focus on the breasts. As you get more experience doing this, you can start to expand your energy and focus on other parts of yourself. The breasts will always be the center, the focal point, the powerhouse of sexual energy and orgasmic potential. But once the energy spreads from there and moves out to contain other parts of you, explore those other parts as well.

Always remember that what you focus on expands. So, if after you've been focusing on your breasts you start to feel a strong vibration in your vagina, investigate that by offering it your attention. Or you might feel something in the crook of your elbow or your neck—a kind of deep erotic sensation that overtakes you. Breathe and put your focus there for a bit, and see what happens. Play with the energy, and give it opportunities to expand and make itself more deeply known to you.

By going with the moment and allowing the pleasure to dictate your focus, you're able to fully inhabit your body and allow your senses to take over. Use your breasts as a starting point and go from there.

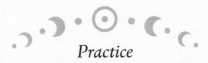

Practice

Drop the Expectation of Orgasm

Expectations define our masculine-driven culture. Many of us approach things like relationships, careers, and sex with expectations about how things should work out. We have expectations about how our partners should act, and the kinds of things we expect them to do to make us feel loved. Children can feel burdened and annoyed by the expectations we have of them to behave and to achieve. When we start a new opportunity—like a new job or career path—we have expectations about what it's going to look like.

When it comes to sex, the heaviness of our expectations for orgasm hangs over the entire act, making it impossible to find the kind of deep, wild pleasure our bodies and spirits are truly yearning for.

Dropping expectations during sex opens up a whole range of potential. It says, "To hell with the end result," and embraces the moment.

Besides, why waste your time straining to build up to one subpar orgasm, when you can actually hold the sensation of a deeper, more expansive orgasm in your body for as long as you want? And even after sex, that expansive orgasm is something you take with you, something that burrows itself into every particle of your body to be used and expressed out into the world around you. All this is possible by releasing expectations.

Clinging tightly to our expectations sets us up for conventional sex. And conventional sex creates conventional orgasms. The kind of orgasms that leave you feeling as if something is off after sex is over. Have you ever experienced this? Being so wrapped up in the act of lovemaking, and tensing your body up to force out that release; and then the release happens, and it's kind of like, *that's it?!*

The one moment of orgasmic release brings your genital area some sensation, and then it's gone. Just like that. Your expectation might have been fulfilled, but not in the way your wild and expansive heart truly deserves.

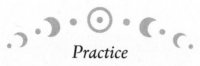

Practice

Only When You're Ready

Receiving your partner inside of you can be uncomfortable when you aren't fully ready for it. Women's bodies need time to drink in orgasmic sensation. We need to feel fully relaxed, at ease, and present before we're able to warm up and receive our partners.

This doesn't have to be some long-drawn-out situation. It's different for every woman. A lot of us struggle with frustration at not being able to feel present enough, or wet enough, or ready enough. This can lead to pain or discomfort when a partner tries to enter us, and can completely disconnect us from our bodies. If we have a male partner, we might get frustrated by his ability to quickly "get hard" and be ready to penetrate. Since we want to please our partners, we might even allow them to enter before we're really ready.

But you can start honoring yourself by being intentional about when you take your partner inside of you. You can start honoring yourself by telling your partner you're not ready, if you don't feel ready.

Your sexual power is not just in your womb, your
vagina, and your breasts. It is in your voice, also.

For some of us, our truth has been buried inside our bodies. We must wake our bodies up by expressing that truth. Know that your truth is powerful, and that you have a right to express it.

When we're young girls growing up in the world, many of us are told not to make waves. We're told to be nice and polite; to smile, even when we're not feeling it. Many of us have tried to conform to this at the expense of our truth. This mindset that culture has prescribed to us has affected our sex lives.

Since many women are natural givers, we also naturally want to please our partners. We want them to be sexually satisfied and fulfilled. But we cannot fully give them that deep satisfaction unless we, ourselves, are truly satisfied. By using our voice to express what we want during sex, we're allowing our partners to know who we are and what we desire. This doesn't only have to apply to letting your partner know whether you're ready to be entered or not. It can also apply to how you like to be touched. Your partner might think that by pulling on your nipple really hard, they are really turning you on; and even though it's kind of uncomfortable for you, your partner seems to be enjoying it, and so you keep your mouth shut.

But the more you keep your mouth shut, the more you withhold your truth. Doing this creates distance and boundaries, not just between you and your partner, but between you and your own body as well.

Whenever something doesn't feel good to you, use your voice. Not in an angry or mocking way. Use it with love. Let your partner know how you like to be loved. This will deepen pleasure for both of you.

By saying you're not ready, you amplify your voice and give yourself the opportunity to stand in your full sexual power.

The next thing you might be wondering is how exactly you can be ready to fully receive your partner inside of you. Taking some of this wisdom here—being in your breasts, slowing down, letting go of tension, and releasing expectation—will help warm your body and prepare you for receiving your partner. Once that happens, you'll know you're ready. The muscles in your vagina will relax and soften. You'll feel the core of your being surrendering into a deep state of reception.

That first moment of taking your partner inside of you must be done with deep intention. Be fully present to the sensation of your partner entering you. Feel your partner's touch against your vaginal opening, and then follow that sensation as your partner moves deeper inside of you. Staying present to the sensation, to your partner's movements, will allow you to feel more pleasure.

Remember that even subtle pleasure is laced with pure power. Try not to skip past feeling into those subtle sensations. Recognizing those sensations, and then giving your full attention to them, will amplify them and deepen orgasm. Bring your presence to each vibration, each sensation, and each fluttering as if they were the only things in existence.

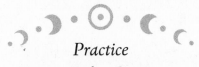

Practice

Involve Your Partner

As your partner is the one you're having sex with, it makes total sense to include them in this new way of approaching lovemaking. If you don't feel comfortable bringing them into the mix yet, take your time with it. Start out by incorporating these changes for yourself, and then once you feel ready, let your partner know about what you're doing.

If your partner is interested and wants to know how they can be involved, you can start off by asking them to be very slow and intentional with their movements. You can also ask them to make time to pay attention to your breasts, to caress them and massage them gently. It's essential to remember that in order to stir up sexual energy in your breasts, the key is not to be so rough. Have your partner go slow and gentle, especially around the sensitive nipple area. Overstimulating the nipples dilutes all the sexual energy in the breasts. But gentle caressing of the nipples and surrounding areas can help spread the energy of orgasm. Experiment with this, and see where the sensations take you.

Having your partner along for the ride means they will also start to reap the benefits of more sensation, pleasure, and orgasm. These slight shifts can wildly transform your sex life, while strengthening your relationship with your partner at the same time.

Practice

Don't Fake Orgasms

Faking orgasms disrupts our own inner alignment with truth. When you're more aware of your body and allowing your sexual energy to find its expression, there's no need to fake orgasms. Becoming orgasmic

supersedes the inclination to go around searching for orgasm or struggling to mechanically go through all the proper steps to bring it on. You
honor your body when you act in accordance with how you're feeling.
Being aligned in this way brings a sense of power and self-love.

Remember: Pleasure Starts Within

Pleasure is not something you seek outside of yourself. And it isn't
something your partner dictates. It's a natural vibration that lives
inside of your beautiful body. It's the definition of *home*. When you
can come home to your body, to your inner wisdom, to your irrepress-
ible power, you *become* pleasure. Everything within you is lit up by it.

Then the orgasmic sensation taking root *inside* of you can begin
to grow and expand its reach to everything *outside* of you.

The body isn't meant to be mechanically induced to bring about
orgasm. I mean, you could do it this way, if you want to stick to the
same old thing you've always known. But knowing that another path
exists—one that is in fierce rhythm with the pulse of life that flows
through you—why not dare to traverse it?

CHAPTER 13 TAKEAWAYS

- Your body has the ability to experience deep multi-orgasmic pleasure.
- Conventional sex limits the potential of what we can experience. It
  is based on tightness, hardness, and mechanical movements. These
  things limit orgasm to the genital area and actually decrease the
  amount of pleasure that can be felt.
- Deep sexual fulfillment must always start with the self. Once you're
  able to harness it and cultivate it within, you can start experiencing a
  deeper kind of sex with your partner.
- Being present to your breasts during sex is a way of starting to liberate the orgasmic potential inside of you.

- During sex, relax into your body. Slow down and be conscious of your breathing. This will support you in allowing yourself to naturally relax into orgasm and allow that feeling to expand throughout the body.
- A woman's sexual power is also in her voice. Use your voice to express yourself and let your partner know what you want during sex.

Chapter 14

PREGNANCY AND CHILDBIRTH

"Birth profoundly changes people—socially, spiritually and psychologically.
All who participate in birth, not just mothers, are affected by its power."
  —Pam England and Rob Horowitz[30]

When a woman becomes pregnant, everything changes. Her womb becomes her focus, the central force around which everything else orbits. Her life becomes defined by her growing belly.

Baby is ten weeks, now twenty, now thirty ...

Pregnancy milestones give her a sense of accomplishment, allowing her to feel just how close she is to meeting her precious baby.

The womb is nothing short of a miracle, working around the clock to carry, sustain, and grow an entire human being.

Pregnancy is a highly spiritual time. It's an opportunity to slow down, to tune in, and to connect to the magic of life blooming within you. It's a sacred time of caring for yourself and doing what is in alignment with soul and body. Instead of allowing the masculine way of action and striving to define who we are, pregnancy can put us in the zone of reclaiming our own natural rhythms.

While nurturing a life inside of us, we must be gentle with ourselves and work on cultivating a deeper sense of self-love. Nurturing ourselves allows

---

30. Pam England and Rob Horowitz, *Birthing from Within* (New Mexico: Partera Press, 1998), 86.

us to nurture the babies we are growing within. Our babies, attached to us by the umbilical cord, are not only able to receive nourishment and oxygen from us; research shows that babies also take on our emotions while they're in the womb.[31]

Pregnancy is the time to lay down all the negative thoughts and disempowering patterns so you can embrace the beauty of what you are. Your baby's well-being depends on it.

The sacredness of pregnancy is something many cultures, over time, have known and acknowledged. Women's bodies change so rapidly during this period. Our wombs and hearts fill up with so much love and joy. We have an opportunity to rest in these feelings and allow ourselves to freely be who we are, without the need to explain or self-criticize.

I cherished both of my pregnancies, because I could not only feel that deep connection to my little ones, but I could also feel a deep kind of connection to all things and people. It was like my own personal womb was being plugged in to some kind of universal womb. Pregnancy taught me to cherish my own natural rhythms and to fall in love with the miracle that is my body.

When you're pregnant, there's nothing left to do but surrender. Surrender to the process, to the mystical cycle of life unfolding within your body. Melting into a state of surrender, becoming soft and receptive, is a reclaiming of our deep feminine truths. Pregnancy puts you smack dab in the middle of your innate wisdom, calling you to pay attention to the sacredness of what you are, and of what you are birthing into life.

Make time to honor your womb during pregnancy, for it is truly doing the deep work of creating life, while also sustaining you and your emotions, moods, sexual energy, and creative flow. If you're pregnant, make an effort to consciously place your hands over your womb—not just to connect with your baby, but to also connect to the source of power that is nurturing you both.

---

31. Miyuki Araki, Shota Nishitani, Keisho Ushimaru, Hideaki Masuzaki, Kazuyo Oishi, and Kazuyuki Shinohara, "Fetal response to induced maternal emotions," *The Journal of Physiological Sciences* 60 (February 2010): 213–220, https://jps.biomedcentral.com/articles/10.1007/s12576-010-0087-x.

Whatever we do consciously, we infuse with great love.

Showering our wombs with attention is a way of demonstrating love, amplifying healing, and flexing our self-care muscles. The truth is, many of us aren't taking care of ourselves the way we should be. During the time of carrying a baby, self-care should become an essential part of our days—and something we continue to do, even after our babies are born. Let pregnancy be that nudge you need to remind you of the essentialness of caring for yourself.

Although being pregnant can sometimes bring physical discomfort, morning sickness, and many different changes to our bodies, it is a time of celebration and abundance. As a pregnant woman, you are in your fullest power; the expression of an ultimate Creatrix in full-fledged physical form. The womb's energies are at their creative peak. Sensuality and emotions may feel amplified at times. Intuition is also heightened during pregnancy, so women should carve out the time to go within and listen to those inner voices.

During pregnancy, women's mental, physical, spiritual, and emotional bodies are alight with potential. It's a great time for visioning, manifesting, and getting clear on what your desires are. Since self-care during this time is of utmost importance, it might be a good idea not to push things too forcefully into fruition. Use this time to get clarity and to fine-tune your visions. However, if you do feel motivation and inspiration pushing you forward into action, by all means, take action. Just be sure to stay aligned to your core, and to listen to what it is your body and heart truly need.

The sacred time of pregnancy is such a fleeting time in a woman's life. Coming back to our bodies during this time is a gift we can give ourselves and our wombs as transformation and new life pulse inside of us.

CHILDBIRTH

When we bring our focus and presence into the act of birthing, we're working in alignment with the wisdom of the womb. Our bodies know this work, deeply, and require our mental focus to propel the experience to the next level. Remember that whatever we do consciously, we infuse with love. Presence is love. Intention is love. When a woman brings her deep concentration into her womb, into the process of birthing her baby, she is offering one of the greatest gifts imaginable.

If all of us were more conscious in childbirth, we could help birth babies who feel loved, safe, and protected. Working in alignment with the womb imbues the baby with a certain kind of ease and joy that is palpable.

A disconnected birth, one where we are distracted and not in alignment with our bodies, will undoubtedly have an impact on our babies and how they feel when they first emerge. The thing is, birth can be hard! It's a beautiful process, but it can also be intense and challenging. This is why there are many women out there who have had feelings of being disconnected while giving birth. If you've experienced this disconnect, know you're definitely not alone. Trust that you showed up in the best way you could in the moment, and that your baby was birthed perfectly.

We can't control all the details of how life will go. When I gave birth to my first child, I experienced a whole lot of disconnect. I was suddenly being whisked away to the operating room for a C-section I did not want. I felt like a total failure, like my body wasn't strong enough to have the "perfect" natural birth I yearned for.

But guess what? Despite feeling that sense of disconnect, despite the birth not going as I had planned…I had a beautiful, healthy baby in my arms at the end, and *that was what mattered*.

Babies spend so many weeks in darkness, bathed in the comfort of the womb. A feeling of oneness with Mama and womb gives babies a sense that all is right in the world and as it should be. After being steeped in that womb comfort for so many months, it can be jarring for a baby to be birthed into the world, regardless of whether or not a woman is able to stay connected during the process.

As mamas, we can do what we can to try to stay conscious as we birth our babies, but we must also be loving and gentle to ourselves when it isn't possible to birth in the ways we want.

The birthing process shows the womb operating at the full height of its power. It can be a long, challenging, painful journey that seems never-ending. But the pain is there, to bring us back to ourselves and to our wombs. The pain is a reminder of our power. It is forcing us to notice just how sacred, badass, and dynamic we truly are.

But many of us choose to medicate our pain to distance ourselves from the messy, hard work of labor. We crave the fast comfort of the epidural. Some of us opt to go without the meds. Know that there is no right or wrong way here. The important thing is to try to stay connected to your body and womb as things are unfolding, and if circumstances make it so you can't stay connected, just go with it. Honor where you're at, and let things happen the way they need to.

If you're pregnant, or you ever become pregnant, be sure to carve out some time to really reflect on what you want your birth to look like. And if you find that you do want to experience a natural birth, come up with a plan to make it happen.

I birthed my second baby naturally, without an epidural, despite having had a C-section with my first. That time around, I had a doula, who was instrumental in helping me have the natural birth I so desperately wanted. Pushing that baby out and feeling every sensation of his birth is forever embedded in my heart. It was one of the most exhilarating experiences of my life. I was so fully in the moment, so present and awake to my womb, that the sensations didn't even register as pain.

I understood then that when we numb the womb, we numb the wisdom available there. That innate power becomes dulled, and our bodies fall out of step with their natural inclination toward birth. I could feel that power, that wisdom, moving through my body as I naturally birthed my second child. It is an experience I will never forget.

Our wombs know exactly what to do. We just have to *trust*. We've got to follow their lead and allow for the magic to work through us. Being present to our wombs during the birthing process is a gift we not only give to ourselves, but to the babies who are being born as well. Again, whatever it is a woman chooses to do—a natural birth or one with an epidural—is the perfect choice for her and her baby. If you're going to be giving birth, remember to try to stay completely present to your womb. Breathe, be in your body, focus on the life emerging from you. Let yourself be alive to each moment. All of it is precious. All of it is part of your sacred womb journey.

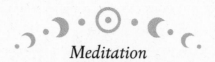

Meditation

Pregnant Mama Mindfulness

This is a great meditation practice to do throughout pregnancy. It will connect you with your little one, as well as to the wonder that is your womb and body. It will also support you in nurturing yourself during pregnancy. You can do this at any stage.

Find a comfortable place to sit, or you can lie comfortably on your side, if that feels better for you. Place your hands over your womb. Close your eyes and start to breathe, dropping your attention into your body.

Next, inhale through the nose, and imagine that breath is being sent down to your baby. Imagine the breath contains all your love.

As you exhale, imagine that breath is gently caressing your baby, infusing them with all your love.

Continue to repeat this for a few minutes.

Chapter 14 Takeaways

- Pregnancy is a very spiritual time. It's an opportunity to slow down, nurture yourself, and listen to your body.
- Our emotional health is of utmost importance, as babies in the womb take on all the emotions we experience each day.
- A pregnant woman has heightened visioning and manifesting powers. Pregnancy is an optimal time for getting clear on plans and goals. But remember not to put too much pressure on yourself to force things into fruition.
- Being more conscious of our wombs and bodies during childbirth supports our babies in feeling safe and supported as they come out into the world.

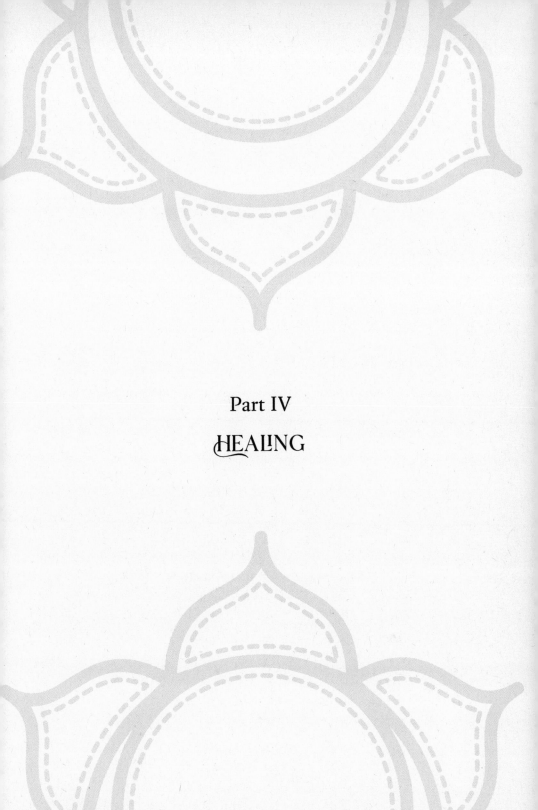

Part IV

HEALING

Chapter 15

MISCARRIAGE AND BABY LOSS

"Life need not be long-lived for it to be meaningful."
—*Unknown*

The day I miscarried, I felt as if my heart had shattered into a million pieces.

It was the second time I had gotten pregnant. Our first son, Benny, was two at the time. And my husband and I were beyond thrilled to be welcoming another child into our family.

I'll never forget that day.

We were living in Los Angeles, and I had a workshop scheduled for the afternoon. I was going to lead a women's circle at Follow Your Heart, a vegetarian restaurant in Canoga Park. It was about ninety minutes before the workshop was going to start, and I was at home, getting ready.

However, something just wasn't right.

I felt my stomach start to tighten, and then cramp. Placing both hands over my womb, I took a breath. *Was everything okay in there?*

My body hunched over, I slowly made my way to the bathroom. As I walked past my husband, he could tell something was off. He asked me if I was all right. I shut myself in the bathroom, muttering something about being fine.

Slowly, I pulled my pants down, and then looked at my underwear. There was blood—something no pregnant woman ever wants to see. I was eleven weeks along, and had been inching my way closer and closer to that safe zone of fourteen weeks—that time when the threat of miscarriage is mostly behind you, and you can start letting friends and family know you're expecting.

But now, with the blood, *I just knew.*

And when I told my husband, he knew, too.

We raced to the hospital, praying we were wrong. Hoping for a doctor to change something, or at least give us a simple explanation as to why it happened and why we shouldn't worry.

In the car ride to the hospital, I called Follow Your Heart and cancelled my workshop. I also called my parents and told them about what had happened. Their concern on the other end of the line was palpable.

A few hours later, after a test and consulting with a doctor, our worst fear was confirmed: I had miscarried the baby.

In the days that followed, that loss burrowed itself deep within my cells, filling me with an emptiness I had never known. Out of habit, I fell asleep at night with my hands on my womb. I woke up, and again, out of habit, my hands would go to my womb. It was still hard to accept that there was no longer a life growing there. At some moments, I even found myself foolishly thinking that there was a chance the baby could still be in there: *What if they were wrong? What if, by some miracle…?*

But I knew this was reality. I felt the difference. When there was life in my womb, I could feel the energy of that life, the spark of it, spinning inside of me. After the miscarriage, I felt a barren, empty field of nothingness. It was like my womb had died as well. It felt lifeless, devoid of any kind of energy.

For every woman who has ever experienced a miscarriage, stillbirth, or the death of a baby, there aren't any words in existence that can possibly fill up that hole that has been created within you. To carry life in the womb, and then to suddenly lose that life, is one of the most devastating feelings in the world. Our babies, growing in our wombs, are literally part of us. And they remain part of us, even after we lose them.

I remember in the weeks that followed my miscarriage, I wanted to stay strong. I had moments when I felt a little ashamed of myself for being so sad.

I would tell myself, *Well, this is something that so many women have experienced. Miscarriage happens in about a quarter of pregnancies. It's common. So get over it.*

But I couldn't deny how I felt.

When the doctor sent us home empty-handed after confirming the miscarriage, I couldn't help but feel cheated. After my pregnancy with my firstborn, the hospital had given me all these pamphlets and guides, overflowing with information on how to care for my new baby. They even threw in a nice backpack for carrying all the materials.

After the miscarriage, I got nothing. No glossy pamphlets with information on what I had just been through, and what to expect in the days ahead. No list of resources for me to reach out to. Just a sad, comforting look in the doctor's eyes, before he left the room and wished me and my husband well.

Nobody likes to focus on baby loss. Maybe it makes us feel too helpless; maybe our world just wants us to move on, to bury ourselves in the task of "trying again."

Our friends and family all mean well when they tell us to try again, in response to our tears. But sometimes a suggestion to try again can make us feel like our pain shouldn't be fully felt.

Every woman navigates pain, loss, and grief in her own way, and in her own time. There is no right or wrong way of doing this. Know that if you suffer a loss, and you choose not to feel the heartache now, it will still be there for you when you are ready to feel it.

It seems that just about every woman has been told or given the indication that her emotions have been too much to handle at some point in her life.

As women, our deepest gifts lie in our ability to feel our emotions fully.

Emotion informs movement, love, and creation. It is a powerful force that can be used to deliver massive impact to the world.

But, as women, we've been told that we're too much. That our emotions are out of control, or crazy, or not tethered to any kind of meaningful reality.

Since emotions are associated with the feminine, this is why there's such a taboo around men expressing themselves and feeling anything. Little boys are told to suck it up, and that if they cry, that means they're acting "like a girl." As if being a girl is so negative and weak.

But woman, let me tell you, your emotions are far from weak. They contain your power; they are part of what makes you who you are. So, when you experience the loss of a baby, or any other kind of loss that completely devastates you, your emotions are there to guide you, to be expressed. The more we can make space in our lives to feel the pain, grief, and heartbreak, the more we can heal. The more we can open up to accepting what is and finding a path forward.

I gave myself the time I needed to heal from my miscarriage. My expression of grief was a way of honoring what I had lost. It was a tribute to the baby I would never get to meet. My pain was all I had left after that blood leaked from my womb that day. And so, I spent many nights sobbing—sometimes alone, sometimes with my husband. I took a painting class for the first time ever, and I painted a mandala to express the grief pressing on my heart. I journaled about it. I reached out to friends when I needed to. I got hugs from my two-year-old, who, daily, came up to pat my belly and say, "Baby. Bye-bye."

Some women who've miscarried feel disappointed in themselves, as if their bodies are lacking somehow, as if something's wrong with them. But this simply isn't true. Our bodies are beyond perfect, magical, and powerful. However, we must accept that sometimes things are out of our control. Sometimes things don't go the way we planned.

Despite this, we must have love for ourselves. We must accept our losses when we're ready to. We must embrace what we have and move forward the best way we know how.

If you've ever miscarried, you know the pain that brings. The disappointment. The grief, the sadness, the frustration. The worry that you'll miscarry again and again, should you try to get pregnant in the future.

A couple of months after my miscarriage, my husband and I decided to try again for another baby. On our first try, I got pregnant. And in the days that fol-

lowed, I started to feel it again. That spark. The excitement of new life blooming inside of me. At the same time, I was still healing from the miscarriage, and
a bit fearful that something would happen to this baby, too. But the pregnancy
went smoothly, and my second beautiful boy, Henry, came into the world. I
cannot tell you what a relief it was to hold my healthy baby in my arms after all
that worry.

As women who have been blessed with the awe-inspiring ability to carry
and give life, we also have to sometimes wrestle with the other side of that coin.
Where there is the potential to create life, there is also the possibility of loss.

When a woman experiences a miscarriage or the loss of a baby, she might
start to believe she isn't good enough. That her body's simply not able to do
the "normal" things it's supposed to do. It's easy to buy into this whole idea of
not working right, or not being able to live up to the expectations of what a
woman is supposed to be and do.

But here's the thing: no matter what struggles you're facing, you are always
worthy and complete. A miscarriage is not a failure. We might be seduced
into thinking it is, due to the fact that there isn't a whole lot of conversation
about miscarriages happening in the world.

After my miscarriage, I had this yearning in my heart for nurturing and healing. As I navigated the next day, and the next one after that, I scoured the internet for resources, for ways to move past this. I didn't know what I was looking
for, exactly, but I figured I'd know it when I saw it.

Well, I never did see it.

But I was able to get through that time with support from my husband.
We were able to talk to each other, to cry about it, to express pain over what
we had lost.

Far too often, our world brushes the topic of miscarriage under the rug.
Like it's not all that important. It's as if the fact that it's common makes it an
unimportant issue.

But that's simply untrue. The life we carried, no matter how brief, was
not unimportant. It was everything.

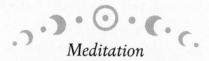

Meditation

Healing Miscarriage, Stillbirth, or Infant Loss

If you've experienced a miscarriage, a stillbirth, or the loss of an infant, use this meditation for support and healing.

Find a comfortable and quiet place to lie down.

Put a blanket over yourself, if you feel you need one.

Get on your side and wrap your arms around your body, giving yourself an embrace. Bring your knees up toward your chest into a comfortable fetal position.

Now close your eyes and focus on the center of your womb. Allow yourself to melt into this space as you take womb breaths.

Give yourself permission just to be. Stay present to the experience of your womb space. Giving our wombs all our attention and our focus naturally brings forth healing. Being present to what is transpiring in this space is all that's required.

When you feel ready to end the meditation, take a moment to whisper words of gratitude for your baby, for the life you carried inside of you. Say anything you would like to express to your baby.

To end the practice, embrace yourself even more tightly. Inhale; as you exhale, sigh out your breath.

Healing isn't a linear experience. It's messy, spontaneous, and unpredictable. Our emotions might come out in waves one day, and the next day, we might feel numb all over. All of us process our pain differently. And through the practice of simply being present to your womb, you can allow your body to do the healing it needs to do.

As you do this practice, you are giving yourself over to what is present in your body, without interference from the mind. Stay with your breath, and with your womb. Let that be enough. And see what comes from it. Allow your emotions to move through you as you keep your arms wrapped around yourself.

Other Ways to Heal

No matter what happens, know that the sun will always be there to greet you each day. Find comfort in the simple things. Take healing baths full of crystals and herbs. Gently massage your pelvis and your womb. Drink lots of water. Be out in nature. Get at least seven to eight hours of sleep. Eat healthy foods that bring vitality into your body. Shower yourself with all the love and care you can.

The highest form of self-care is paying attention to our feelings and emotions. Instead of tightening, find ways to soften into the pain pressing into your heart, or the heavy weight in your stomach. In the long run, know that it is more painful to force the pain away than it is to simply sit with it. All on your own time, of course. Listen to your body and your heart, and they will show you the way forward.

Chapter 15 Takeaways

- Our emotions are part of our natural gifts and are calling for us to feel each one of them fully—whenever we're ready.
- Our wombs are in need of love, attention, and healing after miscarriage or baby loss. Make time to be present to your womb and to care for yourself.

Chapter 16

HEALING FROM SURGERY

"Surgery is not a failure, but a healing opportunity."
—*Christiane Northrup*[32]

In my lifetime, I've had three abdominal surgeries. The first was my C-section in 2011. The other two surgeries, which occurred in 2018 and 2022, happened as a result of the scar tissue created by my C-section.

Before my cesarean, I had never heard anything about how detrimental scar tissue could be. There was no mention of scar tissue on the surgical consent form. Nobody spoke of the impact, the potential damage that can be done to the body.

Scar tissue is the body's way of trying to heal whenever it is cut into during surgery. It can also be created from injury. What happens is, the tissues on the inside become tough and tangled; they start to grow and form sticky adhesions that spread across the fascial layer of the body. When this happens, the body can fall out of balance. You might start to experience pelvic pain, abdominal pain, tightness, or numbness. Your tissues and organs might stick together. You might experience bowel obstructions, bloating, or nausea. In my case, I experienced a pretty severe bowel obstruction. My small intestine got caught on my scar tissue and started to get all twisted up.

---

32. Northrup, *Women's Bodies, Women's Wisdom*, 819.

As I mentioned earlier in the book, the scar tissue caused my small intestine to tie into a tight knot. The pain was about one hundred thousand times greater than natural childbirth, and unfortunately, that's not an exaggeration! It felt like death. I *literally* thought I was going to die. Luckily my surgeon got to it in time, before all the tissue in my intestine died out. If he hadn't operated on me when he did, I wouldn't be alive today.

I'm grateful he was able to save my life, even though surgery was what created this mess in the first place. The problem is that every time a new surgery is performed, more scar tissue is created in the body. The other problem is that every doctor I've spoken to—at least six of them—has told me that nothing can be done to break down scar tissue, and that this is just a problem I'll have to live with for the rest of my life.

In 2022, I started experiencing bowel obstructions again, but not as severely as the first time. This time, my intestine twisted and got stuck on the scar tissue, but it didn't end up in a knot. It was still severely painful. A new surgeon had to operate in order to reach in and snip out the scar tissue causing the problem. I'm now six months out of surgery—and more determined than ever not to go back.

I've become obsessed with finding ways of breaking down my scar tissue. Despite what doctors have said, there are so many amazing people out there who are doing the work of helping others soften scar tissue from previous surgeries. Some physical therapists are using visceral manipulation to support their clients in tackling the scar tissue head-on. Others are using electric microcurrent therapy and even laser therapy to break down scar tissue.

I've explored microcurrent therapy and visceral manipulation, which have both helped my scar tissue tremendously. I've also been spending time in the infrared sauna and using castor oil therapy to help with my scar tissue. If you've ever had surgery, look into the ways in which you can work with and break down your own scar tissue so that it doesn't become a problem over time. Some women experience problems with scar tissue within months of having surgery; for others, it might take a decade or even longer to notice the impact scar tissue has had on the body. And other women will be fortunate enough to never experience any of the harmful effects of scar tissue.

I wish someone had told me a long time ago about the importance of breaking down my scar tissue. Having armed myself with so much knowledge now, I've been doing everything I can to heal my belly and womb from the trauma of surgery.

Many of our wombs have been subjected to surgery, and some of it has been medically unnecessary. A 2015 study shows that almost one out of five hysterectomies may not have been necessary to perform.[33]

Aside from C-sections and hysterectomies, some women have experienced the surgical removal of cysts or fibroids, or the removal of the ovaries or other reproductive organs. No matter what kind of surgery it is, it's a jarring experience for the body to endure.

I've struggled to heal, and to love my body after each of the three surgeries I've had. Not only that, but I've also felt that sense of distance, of not intimately knowing my body like I used to. Surgery creates so many changes that it can be challenging to bring our bodies back into balance and harmony.

After you've experienced surgery, it's important to go slow, to give your body the time it needs to heal and recover. Once you're able to start feeling physically better, you can go about the work of healing your body emotionally and spiritually. It can be as simple as taking some time each day to place your hands gently over the area that was operated on, and just breathing. Sometimes we want to push forward and forget about all our body has endured. But when we take the time to show our body some love, to acknowledge what it's been through, we're able to heal ourselves more deeply.

In our world, we often place our attention on the exterior. We're obsessed with what the scars on the outside look like, but we neglect to consider the healing that needs to take place with our scars on the inside. And I'm not just talking about scar tissue. I'm also referring to those internal scars, those emotions and energies that are unprocessed and tightly locked within ourselves.

33. Susan Perry, "1 in 5 hysterectomies in U.S. may be unnecessary, study finds," MinnPost, January 18, 2015, https://www.minnpost.com/second-opinion/2015/01/1-5-hysterectomies-us-may-be-unnecessary-study-finds/.

If you've ever endured surgery of your belly, womb, or other reproductive organs, know that your body is aching for your attention. It has been through a great deal. It has worked so hard over the years to sustain and nurture you, to keep you alive and vibrant. It does this despite the ways in which we ignore our bodies and opt to live in our heads. It does this despite our refusal to slow down and honor what our intuition is telling us.

The impacts of surgery are not simply over after the incisions heal. There is a deeper healing that needs to take place within, and this is our chance to nurture ourselves and love our bodies, minds, and spirits back into alignment.

As you heal from surgery, know that what has happened to you does not make you anything less than a powerful woman. And if you've had something taken from you—whether it was your womb, your ovaries, your fallopian tubes, your cervix, or your breasts—know that this does not mean you are lacking in any way. You are a strong, brilliant, and wildly capable woman. You are an absolute blessing on this planet. Nothing can change that. Nothing can detract from the light that you are. Accept your body fully, as it is now, because that's where your power lies. That's where your magic is.

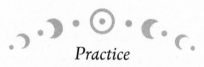

Practice

Healing after Surgery

This is a visualization that can be done anytime after you've had a surgery. Even if it has been years since you've had surgery, I still recommend you do this. It's never too late to heal.

Find a comfortable place to lie down on your back. Place your hands over your lower belly and pelvis.

Take some womb breaths, and just pay attention to this space. Notice what you feel here. Notice if your pelvis or reproductive organs have anything to share with you. Even if certain reproductive organs are no longer physically there, their energy is within, and they can still communicate with you.

After several minutes of listening, take a moment to set an intention. Make your intentions for healing known. Tell your reproductive organs that you are healing them, that you are bringing them back into balance.

Now, on your next inhale, imagine you are breathing a healing golden light all the way down to your reproductive organs.

And as you exhale, visualize the light massaging and healing your reproductive organs.

Continue this breath for at least ten minutes.

When you're finished, rub your hands lovingly over your pelvis and lower belly. Thank your reproductive organs for all they've done for you; acknowledge them for all they've endured.

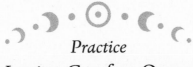

Practice

Letting Go of an Organ

This practice can be done anytime after losing an organ, or multiple organs. You can also do this if you've had to have your breasts removed. The key is to be gentle with yourself during this time and to give yourself the space to grieve this loss.

Get into a comfortable seated position. Alternatively, you can lie down, if you're feeling called to.

Place your hands over the area your organ was taken from.

Take womb breaths here, and if you feel safe to, allow yourself to express any grief or sadness you might be feeling over this loss. There's no time limit on this. Whenever you feel like you're ready, move on to the next part.

Now, leave one hand over this area where you lost your organ. Take your other hand and place it over your heart. Feel the connection between your heart and this area where your organ used to be. Let the love from your heart pour into this space. Take a few minutes to do this.

Finally, tune in to the area where your organ used to be, still keeping your hands in the same positions (one hand over the heart, and one hand over the missing organ). Although the organ is no longer there physically, feel into this area and try to connect with the organ's energy. Feel the energy of this organ still in that space. Feel that energy as vibrant and alive and pulsing with wisdom. Know that this energy is always here for you to tap into, and to seek guidance and love from, whenever you need it.

End this practice by expressing gratitude for your reproductive organs and your sacred feminine body.

Chapter 16 Takeaways

- After any kind of surgery, our bodies need healing, love, and attention.
- If you've had surgery, look into ways to break down your scar tissue so it doesn't cause any problems for you later on. There are so many resources out there, and countless paths you can take: visceral manipulation, self-massage, laser therapy, and microcurrent therapy are all great places to start. In the resources section of this book, I share some links you can look into.
- Even if we've lost certain reproductive organs or our breasts, that does nothing to detract from the fact that we are powerful and amazing women.
- After a surgery, go slow and be gentle with yourself. Shine love and acceptance onto those parts of you that have been operated on. Remember that your body has done so much work to keep you balanced and alive; have gratitude for that.

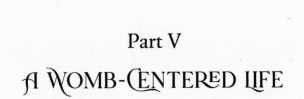

Part V

A WOMB-CENTERED LIFE

Chapter 17

ƒINCESTORS

"The ancestors function as guides, warriors, and healers."
    —*Luisah Teish*[34]

When my dad died in 2015, I experienced a grief unlike any I had ever known. It didn't just feel like he'd been taken away; it felt like an actual physical part of me had been taken away as well. Like I was missing an organ or a limb.

The finality of his death was something I wasn't prepared for. I don't know that any of us are truly ever prepared when someone so very close to us dies.

Around the time of my dad's death, all the electronics in our house went haywire. Clocks just suddenly stopped ticking. An iPad that was perfectly fine just completely died out, never to turn on again. A relative came over to pay his respects, and as he walked through the door, he noticed that his watch completely stopped working.

Days later, I read somewhere that after a person passes, electronic devices might shut down or act funny. The reasoning might be that after a person leaves their physical body, they somehow start to affect electronic energy to let others know they're still there.

---

34. Luisah Teish, *Jambalaya* (New York: HarperCollins, 1985), 80.

To me, at the time, I took these experiences all casually, as mere coincidences. I just felt so much heartbreak and was struggling with how to navigate it all. As spiritual as I had always been, I didn't really have a connection with the idea that life goes on after death. I couldn't allow myself to accept that. When my dad took his last breath, I just figured that a door would shut. That it would close forever, and I would have no access to him.

But in the weeks that followed, as all the messages and signs from my dad started to come through, my mindset began to shift. Life after death became something tangible to me.

I would sit in meditation in my room, and try to communicate with my dad. Every time I waited for a response, I'd feel zaps of electricity shooting through the left side of my body. It was a sensation I had never felt before.

Along with that, my one-year-old was seeing my dad everywhere he went. He'd often point up to the ceiling and say my dad's name. Or we'd be sitting at the table, eating dinner, and he'd wave across the room, greeting my dad. Or we'd be in the car, and he'd indicate that my dad was sitting next to him. All of us tried to look every time, but we couldn't see anything.

This continued for about two to three months, and then one day, there was nothing. My little one stopped seeing my dad everywhere, and I stopped experiencing the feelings of electricity. It was as if my dad was there for a short period of time after his passing to provide comfort, and once he knew things were okay, he took off.

Although my dad's passing was one of the most painful experiences of my life, it was also one of the biggest gifts of my life. To have this confirmation of existence beyond death has changed everything for me. Also, to be able to continue my relationship with my dad, even after he is no longer physically on this earth, has been a true blessing. I no longer feel the electricity through my body when I speak to him, but I do continue to talk to him and to share things that are going on in my world.

Our relationships with our deceased loved ones continue.

Even though we don't have a person's physical presence here with us, even though we can't hear their voice or feel the warmth of their touch, they do live on. And not just as a memory, or something that we keep tucked away in our hearts. Their spirits actually live on, and we can continue to connect with and talk to them whenever we need to.

This is true for all our ancestors, even ones whom we've never known or met. Our ancestors are always part of us. They have laid the groundwork for the lives we're living today. Their struggles, their joys, their hopes and dreams— all of these things are energetically intertwined with who we are.

Some mornings, I'll wake up, fill a special container with water, and leave it on my altar as an offering to my ancestors. I'll say a prayer of gratitude, honoring and acknowledging the lives of my ancestors, letting them know they are not forgotten.

I close my eyes and try to imagine those who came before me over the centuries. I try to feel them, to know their energy. I tell them that my own path, my own healing journey, is for them as well. I know that when I heal, they heal.

This continuing line of life and love is ever evolving. The lives we live today can nourish and heal our ancestors' lives—and the lives of our future great-great-great-grandchildren.

Traditional African practices and religions acknowledge that working with our ancestors is an important piece of the puzzle. It's a way to bring forth healing, transformation, and a deeper connection with all.

You might be wondering: How does the womb tie into all of this, exactly?

The womb is actually the power source that can deepen this connection to our ancestors. As our wombs are places of birth and creation, they connect with all other wombs that have come before them. Think about all the wombs that had to be involved to eventually make you. It wasn't just your mother's womb. It was *her* mother's womb, and before that, it was her *mother's mother's* womb. It took an infinite number of wombs to get to you. There is no greater miracle than that. Look at any person, and think about the infinite amount of wombs it took to get them here as well.

This is how precious life is. This is how connected we all are.

The sustaining energy of the womb has kept our species in motion for centuries. Every womb on this earth is a gift and should be blessed as such. We need to start waking up to the wonder of what we are. Feeling back into your line of ancestors, reaching out to them with love and reverence—this will bring you in full recognition of the power you contain in your every cell.

Work with your womb to deepen your ancestral connections. Know that any healing you do through your womb directly heals your ancestral line. All the many wombs that came before your womb live on inside of you. Your ability to heal, evolve, shift, and grow makes an impact on the lives that existed in this world before you.

Make time to bless your ancestors. Even though you didn't know them in a physical way, they're still here for you. They're part of you.

My relationship with my dad, while he was alive, is one I'll cherish always. The relationship I have with him now, since he has passed away, is one I am so grateful to be able to continue. I feel him and understand him in a deeper way than I could have when he was living. And he also sees me and understands me in a new way than he did when he was here.

If you've shared time on this planet with ancestors whom you personally lost—like a parent, or grandparent, an aunt or uncle—keep the connection alive. They're still here with you. They will never leave you. Your relationship will not be the same as it was when they were here, obviously; it will be different. You will have to get to know them in a whole new way—a way that isn't limited by the physical life you recognize.

ANCESTOR ALTARS

Create an altar for your ancestors so that you can honor and recognize them daily. I have a few different altars in my home—one for honoring ancestors, one for all my crystals, and one general altar where I have something included from each of the four elements. My altars serve as my go-to spots each day for when I want to meditate, set an intention, connect with an ancestor, or do any visualization work.

On my ancestor altar, I keep framed photos of my ancestors, along with some candles and a few special crystals. I try every morning to leave a water offering for my ancestors to show them I remember them. I also place my hands over my heart and say a little prayer for them while expressing gratitude for the lives they lived on this planet.

I would love to say that I do this every day. I try to do it daily. My problem is I have so many practices I love to integrate into my mornings, and sometimes I need to pick different ones to focus on. But I do try to honor my ancestors as much as I can.

Creating your own altar is a simple way of honoring your lineage and healing your womb in the process.

Here are some ideas for what to put on your altar...

- Photos of loved ones who have passed
- Candles
- Incense
- Flowers
- Crystals
- Statues
- A piece of fabric or a scarf
- Paintings or photos of certain figures (like Mother Mary, Oshun, Kuan Yin, or Ganesha)

You can use a small table, a chest, a windowsill, or a bookshelf to set your altar on top of. I usually like to take a beautiful piece of fabric or a scarf and neatly place it on whatever surface I'm using. Then I set up the items on top of the fabric.

Express your creativity, and let your heart guide you toward arranging the perfect ancestor altar for you.

Once the altar is finished, take some time to bless it. Sit in front of it and set an intention. Take a cup of water in your hands and speak positive words about what you hope to experience with your altar. Then dip a few fingers into the water and sprinkle it onto your altar, infusing your new space with your intentions and blessings.

Spend a little time at your altar each day, if you're able to. Make an offering, say a prayer, sit and meditate, journal, or simply stand at your altar and say a heartfelt thank-you to your ancestors. Something as quick as standing at your altar, placing your hands over your womb, and breathing your gratitude into that space is also very healing. It's a quick way of connecting to your ancestors and your womb, while giving yourself a moment of inner stillness. Throw in a womb breath or two, and that's all you need.

Try not to overwhelm yourself with devoting too much time at your altar and with your ancestors. Sometimes we get so excited about trying out new things and bringing empowering habits into our days that we tend to get a little too ambitious with the amount of time and energy we put out.

It's like when New Year's Day rolls around every year. Everyone gets real excited and starts to concoct a whole series of healthy habits they're suddenly going to find the time for. When I was living in Los Angeles, before I had kids, I was at the gym every day, for about two to three hours a day. I used to love the time I had there. But I always braced myself for January.

At the beginning of the year, without fail, there seemed to be an extra three hundred people at the gym, committed to showing up and finally knocking down their health goals for the year. I have nothing against people who want to achieve their health goals, but at the time, seeing them suddenly invade the gym irritated me to no end. However, come February, all the crowds would fade away like clockwork, and things would go back to the way they were. I suddenly had quick access to all the machines and equipment again. I just had to wait it out.

Don't try to take on too much at once. Integrate your ancestor altar into your life in a way that's organic and makes sense for your lifestyle. Women take on so many things day to day. We're balancing careers, kids, partners, and a whole load of other responsibilities. Taking care of our wombs and our bodies, making time to recognize our ancestors, engaging in self-care—all these things can be interwoven into our day effortlessly. By devoting just minutes to feeding our souls and nurturing our bodies, we can refresh ourselves and avoid things like burnout, stress, and overwhelm.

Instead of proclaiming that an hour of your day will be spent doing womb breaths and sitting at your altar, start simple. Build your way to wholeness one minute at a time. This isn't a race. There's nowhere you need to be, other than in this moment right here.

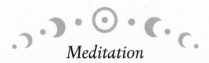

Meditation

Connecting to Your Ancestors

This meditation is all about connecting to all the wombs that worked together to lead to you.

Find a cozy and comfortable place to sit or lie down.

Place your hands over your womb, and, as always, take a few womb breaths to center yourself.

Now, imagine yourself in your mother's womb. Take a couple of womb breaths here.

Then imagine your mother, carrying you in her womb, and concurrently in her own mother's womb as well. Take a couple of womb breaths here.

Now imagine your mother's mother in her mother's womb, and breathe here.

Continue doing this, going back in time and connecting to every mother in the line that came before. You can go back to as many wombs as you like, whether it's five or twenty of them.

Notice how you feel as you do this, as each womb comes in to encircle the wombs that come after it.

Once you're finished, take some time to sit in stillness and be present with whatever feelings come up.

Close things out by feeling gratitude for all the wombs it took to create you.

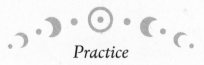

Practice

Ancestor Gratitude

Light a candle on your altar. As your eyes softly focus on the flame, concentrate on the center of your heart. Take a moment to feel all the love, compassion, and energy that vibrate there. Now, either out loud or in your head, say this prayer for your ancestors:

> *Gratitude to my ancestors*
> *To the precious ones who came before me*
> *Your lives mattered*
> *All the joys and heartaches mattered*
> *All of what you were lives on in me*
> *You paved the path*
> *You lit the way*
> *You opened the door*
> *For me to walk through*
> *I honor you*
> *I celebrate you*
> *I cherish you*
> *Please continue to guide me*
> *To show me the way*
> *To bless my path*

CHAPTER 17 TAKEAWAYS

- It doesn't matter whether or not you knew your ancestors physically. They are always here with you to guide and support your life.
- You can connect more deeply to your ancestors by tuning in to the womb space. You are connected to a long line of wombs, which all have contributed to creating your precious life.
- Create an ancestor altar. Start to bless your ancestors. Speak to them. Offer them your love and gratitude. Keep the presence of your ancestors alive in your daily life.

Chapter 18

THE MOTHER RELATIONSHIP

"To describe my mother would be to write about a hurricane
in its perfect power. Or the climbing, falling colors of a rainbow."
                                    —Maya Angelou[35]

Ever since she was young, my mom has been a fastidious saver. I, on the other hand, have spent most of my life spending money the second it came into my hands. In all fairness to myself, as I've grown older, I've been taking saving way more seriously—but it took me some time to get there.

Sometimes I look at my mom and marvel at the fact that I actually came out of her womb. Where my mom is informed by her practical Capricorn sensibilities, I lean in to my Leo-like nature, which is to say that I go wherever my creativity and passion happen to take me.

Although my mom and I are so vastly different, we are remarkably tethered by the deep bond of our wombs. Her womb brought me life. It was within her where I was nurtured into being, within her where I first became acquainted with this precious life I am so grateful to have. It was also within her where my own womb was created.

I know these things are obvious. But sometimes it helps to stop and experience a sense of awe of the things we've become accustomed to in our lives. Feel awe for the fact that you are a woman. Feel awe for your womb and

---

35. Maya Angelou, *I Know Why the Caged Bird Sings* (New York: Random House, 1969), 59.

your body. Feel awe for your mother's womb, and what it took to carry you and birth you.

All of that is part of you. It's part of your story. That story contains many beginnings, one of which is your mother, who possesses the womb from which you came. Regardless of your relationship with her, she is the beginning of you. Her womb bathed you with love and cocooned you in darkness, allowing you to grow and evolve, preparing you for the world outside of her.

It was in her womb where you grew all your organs, all your eyelashes and fingers and toes. It was in her where you basked in the comfort and life-sustaining energies the womb provides. It was in her where you gained firsthand experience of what it's like to be unified, to be one with something other than yourself. You existed in a cocoon of comfort and connection, tied to placenta, womb, and Mom in a deeply beautiful and effortless way.

Your mother's Womb Story is also your Womb Story.

Regardless of your relationship with your mother, she is part of you, and you are part of her. She might be (or if she has passed, *might have been*) the furthest thing from a perfect mother; she might not have been there for you in the ways your heart has longed for. But she is part of you.

The nature of your mother's being is profoundly intertwined with your own. Your mother, her womb—they were your portal into this world. By honoring your mother and her womb, you honor the sacredness of your own being. Take time to feel and express your gratitude for her womb, for the place in which you gestated, and your own womb will flourish.

If you have a strong and loving relationship with your mother, this kind of practice will be easier for you. But if you struggle to see eye to eye with your mother, if you've been estranged from her, if you cannot allow yourself to let go of things she might have said or done in the past, this practice will undoubtedly unearth some pain and heartache for you. You might not be ready to embrace the idea of honoring your mother just yet. Each one of us is doing the best she can, based on the circumstances of her life. No one can know what it's like to have lived through your unique life experiences. You must discern for yourself whether or not you're ready to take this monumental step.

Know that this doesn't require that you cozy up next to your mother. You can honor her womb and express gratitude for her role in bringing you into this world without having to speak to her or be near her. She doesn't need to know you're doing this work.

For women who have never met their mothers, or who have lost their mothers at young ages, you can still work through this practice. It will help you heal some of the sadness that comes with lacking a mother figure for most or all of your life.

Our mothers' wombs can be honored and appreciated whether they've passed or are still alive. Mothers who are no longer on this physical plane will still know and receive the honor and love we send them. They are still here with us, just in a different kind of way. And we can still continue our relationship with the mothers we have lost. By reconnecting to a mother who has passed away, we can bring healing and love not only to the life she once had, but also to her spirit, and to her many future lives.

Since our mothers' wombs housed our own wombs, they are forever linked to us in a way that is unbreakable. This means that when your mom's womb gets love, attention, and healing, your womb does, too. So do the future wombs that come after you.

The deep work we do on ourselves does not exist in a vacuum. When we heal ourselves, we heal other women.

When we forgive ourselves, we give other women the courage to also forgive. When we dare to push our limits, to go outside of our comfort zone, to plunge madly into those areas that interest and excite us, we inspire other women to do the same. Just as we're interconnected with the energies of our mothers, we are also one with the energies of all women. Our feminine power is a shared force that comes from the same creative, electric source. What we do affects all women. Never think that you're alone in this very important work of coming back to your authentic and powerful self. You have legions of women behind you. You're never by yourself in this.

Whether or not it might feel like it in this lifetime, know that your own mother's love is and always will be part of you. Whether or not she has known how to express that love to you, it is there, glowing like an ember inside of her. Maybe it has never been revealed to you in words or gestures, but it's there.

When you're ready, practice coming back to your mother's womb, to the very beginning, to the point where it all started for you. If you can go there, you will find a stillness so intoxicating that it melts you. It might sound crazy, or overly simple, but it's true: your mother's body and womb hold limitless potential for your evolution as a woman in this world.

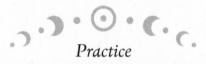

Practice

Forgiving Your Mother

This practice is for women who have had difficult relationships with their mothers. Only do this if you feel you are ready to forgive. And know that by doing this practice, you are by no means opening the door to becoming BFFs if she's still alive and that's not what you want. You can still keep that physical boundary up and do this practice of forgiveness.

Start by sitting up with a straight spine.

Begin to take some womb breaths, and relax your body.

Now, imagine your mother is seated directly in front of you, about two feet away. Make eye contact with her (as you continue to keep your eyes closed). Look deep into her eyes. Look so deep that you can just about see her soul. See her as the vulnerable human she is—someone who is doing the best she can with what she has in the moment. Allow yourself to witness her without the confines of past events or exchanges clouding your mind.

When you're ready, let her know that you forgive her. Mouth the words. Or say them out loud. Or say them in your mind. Whatever feels most comfortable to you. Tell her anything else you feel you need to say. And whatever you do, say it with love.

Then, in silence, hold the eye contact with her a little longer.

If it feels safe for you, end the practice by wrapping your arms around your mother for a celebration hug.

It's not easy to forgive someone who has caused deep pain in your life, especially if that someone has played an integral role in bringing you into the world. It takes some major bravery to do a practice like this. Remember to breathe and be gentle with yourself for the rest of the day.

HEALING YOUR MOTHER'S WOMB

While you were in your mother's womb, you were one with her. All her thoughts, feelings, and emotions—they were part of you as well. You heard the sounds of her voice, her laughter, and all was right in the world. Her womb offered you warmth, comfort, and life.

At the same time, you were in a vulnerable position you had no control over. You had to trust that your mother would do whatever she could to keep you safe and healthy, until the time was right for you to come out into the world and exist outside of her.

For this next practice, you'll be experiencing what it was like to be in your mother's womb. Being carried in the womb was a time in which you were intimately aware of its power. As your first home, it gave you a sense of peace, beauty, and comfort—something we can spend our entire lives trying to replicate out in the physical world.

A big part of our lives is spent searching for ways to come back to those feelings of comfort and oneness we experienced in the womb.

Once we are birthed, there can be so much pain and confusion surrounding accepting ourselves as beings separate from our mothers. As we get older, some of us can tie ourselves up in knots struggling to carve out lives that give us those same feelings we experienced while inside of the womb.

The thing is, we truly don't need to struggle. That sense of being separate from everyone and everything else is all just illusion. Underneath the surface of all things, there is a pulse, a dynamic kind of rhythm or energy that binds all things and all people together. The entire world is a kind of cosmic womb in this regard—a place throbbing with oneness and overflowing with love and protection.

Many of us can't see this, can't hear the rhythm, because we've grown too accustomed to believing there are walls, boundaries, and divisions between us and everyone else. But if we can open our hearts and heal our wombs, we can fall back into step with this rhythm, with this divine alignment. Then we can exist in full acknowledgment of the cosmic womb, which will only deepen and expand our connection to our own wombs.

The first step toward getting there, however, is to find the power of our own wombs again. Once we can fully take ownership of that power, we can start to open up to life in a more organic, rich, and alive way. We can start to come back to ourselves. One of the ways to experience this is to start from the beginning: inside your mother's womb.

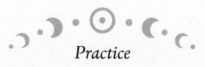

Practice
Mother Womb Healing

Since your mother's womb held your womb, there is some major opportunity here for lots of healing, acceptance, and transformation.

Get into a fetal position. Bring your knees up toward your chest and wrap your arms around them.

Try to imagine yourself back inside your mother's womb. Feel the comfort and security this brings to your body. Just allow yourself to exist in this space without any kind of pressure or expectation.

If you hear, feel, or see something, pay attention to it. Listen to the words your mother's womb has to share with you. It could be something specific about what you experienced while being formed in her womb, or it could even be bringing up the feelings of love you felt while inside your mother. Exist in this place, and let yourself feel whatever is present there for you.

When you can no longer hear or sense that there's anything else you need to know, imagine you are placing your hands over the inside of your mother's womb. Send love and healing energy directly to her womb. Feel that love and healing energy radiating from your hands and into her womb and body.

Spend a few minutes here, and then end the practice when you are ready.

Feel free to write about your experience in your Womb Journal. And know that whenever your mom experiences healing, you are experiencing healing as well. You are both inextricably connected, and this connection cannot fade or ever be eradicated. Her healing is your healing, and, of course, your healing is her healing as well. So, after you do this practice, you might experience your own womb feeling energized.

CHAPTER 18 TAKEAWAYS

- You and your mother, no matter what your relationship is, share a connection that is unbreakable. Your wombs are forever linked.
- When your mom's womb is healed, so is your womb. And when your womb is healed, so is your mom's womb.
- If you've had a difficult relationship with your mother, you can do work to forgive her. But only forgive if you are truly ready for it. Know that forgiving her doesn't mean you suddenly have to welcome her into your life with open arms.

Chapter 19
WOMB SISTERHOOD

"When women circle, we learn to trust ourselves and one another. We step into our sovereignty as individuals while also learning how to be part of a collective."
  —Tanya Lynn[36]

The first time I ever joined a women's circle, I felt as if I had arrived home. Although I didn't know a single woman in the group—and had only spent a mere two hours with all of them—there was this sense of familiarity, of coming back to something I had long forgotten.

During the circle, we lit candles, made affirmations, called in the four directions, and manifested together with deep intention. It was one of the most intimate and highly transformative evenings I had ever had. I remember being in the car, driving home after, and buzzing with excitement over my newfound connections to the other women and, of course, to myself.

When it comes to tapping the limitlessness of our feminine potential, sisterhood is essential. Without sisterhood, there would be a void, an empty space that would be challenging to fill otherwise. Sisterhood offers a respite away from the confines of society's prescribed notions.

---

36. Tanya Lynn, *The Art of Leading Circle* (New Fern Publishing, 2020), 8.

One womb, all on its own, is a powerhouse.
But when many wombs come together, that power is
multiplied exponentially.

Even if women aren't necessarily coming together to make some specific impact on the world, they do this inadvertently by forging their sisterhood.

Women come together over so many different reasons. They form bonds over mutual interests, like cooking, dancing, hiking, or quilting. They might create sisterhood over their desire to improve their lives, whether it's through being more financially abundant, reading more books, or taking their businesses to the next level. They might come together in motivation over some galvanizing purpose, like raising money for the PTA, bringing food and clothes to unhoused individuals, or going door-to-door to help a fellow sister campaign for elected office. Or they might form actual women's circles, where they engage in rituals, create space to hear one another, and find ways to support each other in their growth.

Over the years, as I've looked at the ways in which women all over the world have united, I've seen how positive and life-changing sisterhood can really be.

Yet despite the power inherent in sisterhood, so many women feel separate from other women, and this drives the need to compete against one another. Competing against each other means we're not making space to honor and recognize the beauty, power, and uniqueness of other women. The game of competition we play cuts us off from any chance of having true and meaningful sisterhood in our lives.

Also, in our social media–driven world, it can be easy to stay separate from others. This seems ironic, given the fact that social media is supposed to establish and nurture connections. However, more and more people are feeling isolated, alone, and depressed by consuming social media. It has become a primary focus for many, though the simple fact of the matter is that social media is not real life.

Many women and young girls who consume a lot of social media start to carry feelings of inadequacy within. We start comparing our lives to the lives of other women we see on our feeds, even though they're not accurate depictions of what life really is. Social media isn't the cause of women comparing themselves to others, but it certainly offers a dominant daily avenue for the comparisons to flourish.

Advertisements and commercials also exacerbate feelings of inadequacy in women, often knowing just the right buttons to push to get us to feel as if we're lacking somehow. All those airbrushed photos in magazines drive many women to forever be chasing some illusive fantasy version of themselves that can never truly exist.

This fractures us within, even though we might not realize it. Our minds might not be consciously processing all the disempowering data, messages, and images we're receiving on a day-to-day basis. But our unconscious is wide awake and taking everything in. This inner crippling creates distance not only from ourselves, but from other women in our lives as well. It stirs the pot, making us feel as if we're not good enough. This brings us to feel threatened by other women, and the need to compete starts to assert itself full force.

I'm absolutely wild about cycles and how they relate to us women, but I've got to put my foot down when it comes to the never-ending cycle of listening to messages that disempower who I am and what I can be as a woman.

Stepping away from disempowering messaging and ideas will not only preserve your sense of self, but it will also inspire you to start reaching out to like-minded sisters. You don't play the game anymore of doubting your worth and looking at other women as the enemy. Instead, you start realizing just how much of an impact you can make in the world by simply creating sisterhood with other women.

When you combine your talents and your strengths with another woman's talents and strengths, you double your impact. Your voice becomes twice as loud. Bring even more women into the mix, and you've got yourself a sisterhood that can make absolutely anything happen.

If women don't all look out for one another, who will?

All of us are weaker when women are pitted against each other. When we're gossiping behind one another's backs, or we're harboring feelings of jealousy toward one another, we hurt all women. We hurt *ourselves*.

As women in this world, we desperately need to stand together.

Women who stand together, rise together.

Find your community of like-minded sisters who see you and accept you for who you truly are. Rally around a cause, find a common interest, heal together, or just simply hang out, because you like each other's company.

---

*Move on from people who don't cherish
or value your presence.*

Life is too precious to waste time in relationships that drain you. Set intentions for deeper connections. Open yourself up to the discovery and initiation of new friendships.

And if trusting other women feels like a major uphill battle for you, ask yourself why that is. Look back into your life experiences and try to recall what happened initially. *When did you stop trusting other women?*

Go into that experience and allow yourself to release it when you're ready. Remind yourself that this life is too sacred to hold on to old energies, experiences, and hurts. Breathe into this knowing and make a pact with yourself to move on from the mindsets and blockages that are keeping you from forming deep bonds with other women. Hold your womb with both hands as you do this deep and holy work. Involve your womb in your healing, and make it an active part of your commitment.

Taking the step toward healing the pain that is tied up in mistrust, judgment, and envy of other women will bring about a tremendous shift of energy. It will clear out those inner cobwebs that are holding you back.

Acknowledging and moving on from these feelings allows us to feel ourselves in a whole new way. When we make judgments and criticize other women, we're really just reflecting feelings about our own selves. Thinking that another woman isn't good enough shows we think *we're* actually not good enough. Snubbing a woman for her appearance, or the sound of her voice, or the decisions she makes in her life shows we are actually rejecting certain aspects of ourselves.

Empower and uphold all the women in your life. Treat them as if they were rare and precious treasures. Celebrate with them, laugh with them, cry with them. Cultivate a sisterhood that fills your soul all the way up.

Start a Womb Circle

If you want to truly take things to the next level, consider starting a Womb Circle.

A Womb Circle is a group of women who get together on occasion for healing, conversation, and transformation. The circle would focus on womb-based practices and give women the opportunity to form a sisterhood.

You can use this book as your guide and explore some of the practices together. You can read through chapters out loud and even plan to have discussions on a variety of topics, like sexuality, menstruation, relationships, creativity, or motherhood.

Cultivating a safe space for other women to talk, learn, and grow together is essential for making a circle like this work. And nothing beats having like-minded sisters who are there to support you and cheer you on.

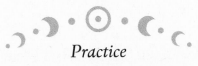

Practice
Cultivating Sisterhood

This is a great practice for connecting your womb to all other wombs in existence. It's about reaching out energetically and feeling that sense of sisterhood among all women. You can do this on your own, or you can even do this with a group of other women in an effort to connect with one another more deeply.

First, sit up with a straight spine and relax your shoulders.

Start to breathe deeply through the nose.

Place both hands below the belly, over the womb space. And continue breathing.

Imagine a line of golden energy extending out of your womb.

Envision that line of golden energy breaking off into many channels and connecting to the wombs of all women. If you're doing this with a specific group of women, then imagine this line of energy is connecting to all their wombs; they should all imagine the same thing.

As you feel this nourishing connection between your womb and other wombs, breathe into it. Stay present to whatever comes up for you in this moment.

After a few minutes, still connected to the other wombs, imagine you are beaming love from your heart, down to your womb, and out through those energy channels to all the women you're connecting with.

Now take a moment to feel love from the hearts and wombs of the other women coming into your body.

Finally, feel love flowing in both directions, from you to them, and them to you; just continue to breathe.

When you feel like you've completed the practice, very slowly allow the lines of energy to disappear. And even though they are disappearing, still allow yourself to feel that lasting connection to other women. Trust that this connection is always there.

The mysteries of the feminine are held in the bodies of every single woman. Although not all of us might be conscious that we carry these mysteries, they're still present there. It's something all women lay claim to. This sacred power is our connection, our lifeline, to one another. We must wield it wisely and with great love.

Chapter 19 Takeaways

- Women thrive when they're part of a sisterhood. One womb on its own is quite powerful. But when many wombs come together, that power increases exponentially.
- Competition and comparison just keep us feeling separate from other women, which also cuts us off from our own personal power.
- Find ways to cultivate sisterhood in your life.
- Start a Womb Circle and bring women together to practice some of the exercises in this book.

Chapter 20

MANIFESTATION

"Whether you are aware of it or not, you manifest things all the time."
—Mystic Dylan[37]

When a woman births a baby into the world, she is revealing something about the power and potential that is inherent in the womb space. She is showing, in a way that is wildly tangible, just how powerful her ability to create truly is.

But the womb's magnificence isn't solely based upon birthing human beings. The womb can also support you in birthing a project, a new business, a work of art, or the paving of a new direction in life.

Don't forget, if it can nurture and birth a whole new person, then it can do just about anything. What we know about the womb and its potential is still in its infancy, due to the fact that we've pretty much only paid attention to the womb as it relates to pregnancy and childbirth.

More than 80 percent of the ocean is currently unexplored, and it's almost as if it's this way with the womb as well.[38] Comparing the ocean and the womb makes sense, as the element of water is associated with the

---

37. Mystic Dylan, *The Witch's Guide to Manifestation* (Emeryville: Rockridge Press, 2021), viii.

38. National Oceanic and Atmospheric Administration, "How much of the ocean have we explored?" US Department of Commerce, last modified February 26, 2021, https://ocean service.noaa.gov/facts/exploration.html.

womb in the ancient chakra system. Our wombs and oceans are full of many mysteries and miracles that haven't been fully comprehended yet.

If you want to manifest something, you can tap into the energies of your womb to support you in making it happen. You have a monumental power source inside of you that is radiating with a ton of potential. Align to your womb, and let it help you create the life you want.

What Does It Mean to Manifest with the Womb?

Manifestation is based on our ability to bring our dreams and visions into tangible reality. It's about actualizing our desires out into the world. Some look at manifestation and think it's simply a way of visualizing what you want, and then sitting back and waiting for it to come to you. But if we all did that, then we'd never get anything done.

*Manifestation is the synchronization
of feeling, intention, and action.*

Although some of us might claim to have no experience in really doing it, we're all manifesting, every second of every day.

The current state of our lives is all hinged upon what we've been manifesting. Our thoughts, our feelings, the way we show up in the world—all of this has contributed to what we're presently experiencing in our lives.

The good news is that if you don't like what you're manifesting, you can make a choice to manifest something else. You can create a life you're absolutely mad for. A life that makes you feel as if you're living smack-dab in the middle of a dream.

Manifesting with the womb is a way to cut through all the noise and chatter and to start realizing your desires. It's a way of stepping into the wisdom of your body and trusting that it will lead you where you need to go.

To manifest with the womb, we must work with two very
essential practices: visualization and embodiment.

Visualization involves being able to create pictures in the mind. Through it, you can imagine every detail of the life you want, or the creation you want to put out into the world. However, if you're solely creating images in your mind, and they aren't really connected to any kind of feeling, your visualization will be superficial and hollow.

That's where embodiment comes into the picture. Embodiment is a way of truly taking on the feelings, emotions, tones, and textures of what you want to manifest and really allowing yourself to feel and experience all of it in your body.

Connecting the powers of visualization to the powers of embodiment makes for a lethal combination. That way, your visualization isn't merely living in your mental universe, which is just a small part of who you are. Instead, it is living in the body—and the womb—filling up the physical, emotional, and spiritual parts of yourself as well. Embodying your visualization locks you in. It puts you in the zone, bringing the experience of whatever it is you want to manifest directly to you.

When that happens, a new kind of feeling is created. It's a feeling of freedom. This is because once you're able to embody the thing, you almost feel as if it's already been manifested. Basically, all the systems of your body have no more need to operate in a state of lack, since the feeling of having manifested is already anchored within you.

Being in this place is powerful. It releases you of any need to forcefully and desperately stalk the fulfillment of the goal or desire. It realizes the goal and desire within you. Then you become attractive to whatever you want to manifest. You become a magnet for it. All the plans you need to make, and the actions you need to take, start coming naturally to you. You don't approach life with a sense of lack or longing. You approach it with open arms and joy, and an attitude that you already have everything you need inside of you.

Practice

Womb Manifestation

Use this practice to start working with your womb in manifesting the life you want. You can do this for anything you want to create for yourself, no matter how big or small.

Find a quiet place to sit.

Before you close your eyes and get settled, think about one thing you want to manifest in your life. It doesn't have to be anything fancy. It could be that you want to have an amazing day, or that you want to have a great meeting at work. If you want to go even bigger, you can think about what you want to create in your life. Pick one thing. Whatever lights you up in the moment.

When you've picked your one thing, place your hands over your womb and close your eyes. Start to take some womb breaths as you let your mind and body relax.

Now it's time to create the visualization in your mind. Whatever you selected, start to form a picture of it in the mind, as if it's already happening. So, if you want to manifest a positive day, see the positive day unfolding in your mind. See what would happen during that day. Take all the time you need to visualize it. This could take anywhere from one to twenty minutes.

Keep taking womb breaths as you visualize.

Now, as you continue visualizing, focus on your womb. Imagine you are placing the visualization in your womb space. It's as if you're taking it out of the mind and just allowing it to sit in the body. Feel the visualization move into the womb.

Now, as you breathe deeply, allow that visualization to expand across the entire body. Instead of seeing a picture now, hone in on the feeling that this picture creates within you, whether it's joy, bliss, peace, comfort, happiness, or anything else. Let yourself feel this in every cell of your body.

Finally, tune in to your heart space and feel the visualization sitting in your heart. Again, there should be no image here—just a feeling. Allow the feeling to be fully present, to fill your heart all the way up.

Don't forget to keep on womb breathing. Do this for as long as you feel comfortable.

When you feel you've completed the practice, take one very deep breath and slowly open your eyes.

Stay aligned and connected to the feeling, even as you open your eyes and come back to the space. Even though you're completing the practice, this is an essential step. You don't want to "snap out of" the manifestation and just casually roll back into your normal day-to-day life. You actually want to bring that feeling you've aligned to out into your life. This will help you "live" your manifestation out in the world.

A Quick and Easy Way to Manifest through the Womb

Pressed for time, but want to build manifestation into your daily life? Or maybe you just want to do it here and there?

The more you practice your manifesting skills, the easier and more effortless it becomes. If you're manifesting haphazardly, when the mood strikes you, you'll find that the results might not be as consistent.

If you're showing up consistently to visualize, embody, and move your dreams forward, you'll find your manifestations will materialize much more quickly.

The truth is, though, many of us are juggling so much every day, and we need quick and simple (yet impactful) ways of manifesting. Having these quick practices are great, because they help us stay consistent.

Quick Practice
Manifesting with the Womb

To unlock your manifesting potential in a short amount of time, try this: place your hands over your womb. State an intention. Make sure to state it in the present tense, like, *I am financially secure.* Or, *I have everlasting love in my life.* When you say those words, either aloud or in your head, imagine that you are planting the words themselves into the center of your womb, like seeds. Repeat these words a few times.

Finally, take a deep breath, and feel the emotion, the vibrancy, the energy of these words resting in your womb. Now, go about your day and just surrender to each moment of it, without trying to control anything.

That's really all it takes. It's an easy way of tuning in to your womb and body and setting the stage for pure magic to take over.

THE DEEPER YOU GO...

As you get more conscious about manifesting, you might notice that you start to become more intentional and aware. Life starts to become more vibrant, rich, and abundant. This is because, as you use the principle of embodiment with your manifestation, you are naturally stirring up the feelings you desire in your body. This puts you in a positive frame of mind and allows you to experience more ease in your daily life. A feeling of completeness may start to wash over you.

During all my years of engaging in the process of manifestation, there's one thing that still amazes me to this day: the deeper I go into embodying my desires, and into being conscious of this precious life I'm creating, the more a kind of intelligence starts to take over. The universe begins to really hear me, without all the distractions in the way. It starts to deliver exactly what my soul desires. It does this effortlessly, without my even having to set the intention for it.

Once you hit this point, you'll know that you're truly locked into a state of flow. It's a beautiful experience when the universe opens up and you surrender to all its magic and mystery. That is the true way of manifesting, when you become so aware and so locked into the universe that you don't even have to think about what it is you want to do or create. The universe seemingly just starts to conspire with your deep feminine energies and brings in all the experiences, opportunities, and people that are for your highest good.

If you don't feel like you can ever get to this point, don't sweat it.

Just remember, we all have our own unique paths in this world. Where you are is perfect for where you are. There's no need to rush or compete or feel as if time has gotten away from you.

Manifestation should be done with a spirit of joy. If we're clenched, desperate, or angry, it simply won't work. The energy has to flow. It all has to be pure. Don't be too attached to what the outcome is.

Fall in love with the process. Fall in love with creating conscious, empowering thoughts about yourself and what you're capable of. Fall in love with designing the most awe-inspiring visions of what you can become; and most importantly, fall in love with what you *already are*.

CHAPTER 20 TAKEAWAYS

- We are manifesting every second of every day, without even consciously putting any thought into it. Once you start being more conscious and intentional about what you want to call in to your life, you can manifest your desires.
- Use feeling, intention, and action to manifest what you want in life.
- Since the womb is the ultimate manifesting power source, we can work with it to create new realities.
- By embodying the manifestation, we allow ourselves to feel it. That feeling reminds us that we already contain everything we need inside of us, and this helps us manifest.
- Remember to approach manifestation with a spirit of joy and not to be too attached to the outcome.

Chapter 21

NOURISHING THE WOMB WITH HEALTHY FOOD

"Green foods will help to connect you to your spiritual essence.
The more green you take in, the more forgiveness comes through."
    —Queen Afua[39]

During my teenage years, I absolutely worshipped McDonald's. While I was in college, my boyfriend (now my husband) and I made constant late-night runs to greasy diners and pizza joints in the city of Boston. However, after we graduated, my boyfriend announced he was going to become a vegetarian.

I'm not going to lie—when I heard his announcement, I was downright pissed. We had bonded so much over our meat-laden diet, and I worried we would lose that connection.

But what could I do? I had to adjust. Within weeks after graduating, we moved into an apartment right off Sunset Boulevard in West Hollywood. I was the cook in our home, so that meant making some shifts in preparing our meals. At first, I would cook separate meals for both of us every day. But then that got to be too much work. So, I decided to start eating vegetarian as well, since it would be easier and save more time to cook the same thing for both of us. As vegetarians, we still ate some dairy, and I had salmon every once in a while.

---

39. Afua, *Sacred Woman*, 86.

Well, after some time, I noticed how pleasurable eating this way was. I started to lose some weight and feel more energy. I didn't realize that switching the way I ate would have such a profound impact on how I felt.

Within several years, I became vegan, choosing to consume no animal products at all. I wanted to take things to the next level. Within days, I started to feel the effects of the diet. I felt as if my body was supercharged. It was seriously unlike anything I had ever experienced. And from there, I never looked back.

Since going vegan, I've felt more clarity, energy, strength, and wellness than I've ever felt in my entire life. I feel lighter, more grounded, and more connected to myself and the world around me. My womb feels nourished and activated. My skin is more soft and supple. And my mind feels radiant and clear. To be honest, I can't even remember what it's like to feel any different. I never in a million years thought I would be vegan, but when I took the plunge, it opened up potential in me I never knew existed.

What you consume impacts the wellness of your womb. Plant-based foods offer many benefits for overall health, wellness, and vitality. Animal products are harder for the body to digest and, in many cases, contain harmful pesticides and hormones that can wreak havoc on the systems of the body. Studies have shown that animal products have a detrimental effect on the body and lead to greater incidents of heart disease and cancer.[40]

Our wombs thrive when they're nourished with healing foods, like vegetables, fruits, whole grains, nuts, and seeds. As our wombs are brimming with the energy of life's cycles, they are in tune with the nature around them. And so, foods that come from nature—that aren't processed—resonate more strongly with the womb.

Now just to make things clear: this isn't a chapter about convincing you to drop everything you know and suddenly become vegan. Ditching all ani-

40. "Red and processed meat linked to increased risk of heart disease, Oxford study shows," University of Oxford, July 21, 2021, https://www.ox.ac.uk/news/2021-07-21-red-and -processed-meat-linked-increased-risk-heart-disease-oxford-study-shows; Jeanine M. Gen-kinger and Anita Koushik, "Meat Consumption and Cancer Risk," *PLoS Medicine* 4, no. 12 (December 2007): e345, https://www.ncbi.nlm.nih.gov/pmc/articles/PMC2121650/.

mal products is a big choice to make, and it might not be the right choice for everyone's situation. If you can even just cut meat and dairy out of your life a few days a week, that would make a big difference in your body and womb. As our world embraces more plant-based options, many people are experiencing the benefits that come with reducing or all-out eliminating their consumption of animal products.

If you're accustomed to eating processed foods and animal products, it might seem daunting to attempt to bring more plant-based, unprocessed foods into your diet. Not only that, but it might sound unappealing in general! Just know that it doesn't have to be all or nothing. As long as you are conscious about looking for ways to bring more plant-based foods into your diet, little by little, your womb and body will thrive as a result.

As a life-generating, creative force, your womb functions best when it's being nourished with healthy, vibrant foods.

Since plant-based foods are cultivated within the earth, they carry the life-sustaining energy of Mother Nature. Eating plant-based foods also further seals the connection between the womb and Mother Nature, allowing for more creative, dynamic, and loving energies to blossom within the body, heart, and spirit.

When we base our diet on processed foods, sugar, and caffeine, the body and womb will suffer. Do you ever notice what your body feels like after you scarf down some fast food or a few cups of coffee? In the moment, it might seem like your body is being infused with a boost of energy, but focus deeper into yourself, and you might notice that heaviness and sludge-like feeling inside of you.

There's a difference in your body when you eat an apple versus when you eat a candy bar. There's a message your body sends you every time you nourish it with healthy, healing foods, and a totally opposite kind of message when you stuff it with junk food.

Food that comes from the earth is drenched in love. It is imbued with Mother Nature's qualities. It contains the energies of the sun, the soil, the wind, and the water. It is full of high-vibrating life force energy, that same energy that resides inside of you. When you fill your body with food that is pulsing with this life force energy, it enhances and nurtures what you are. Those life force energies infuse the womb with even more creative power, love, wisdom, sensuality, and vitality.

Eating nourishing, healing foods is a powerful act of self-love.

Eating healthy is an opportunity you have multiple times a day, a week, a month, and a year. Make the choice to nourish yourself each and every single day. Let the choice to eat healthier, plant-based foods be a gift to yourself.

WHAT TO PUT IN YOUR WOMB

If you nourish your womb and body with more plant-based, unprocessed foods, your health, wellness, and immunity will be supercharged. You'll have more energy and clarity. The systems in your body will move into harmony and balance. Fill your womb with fresh and vibrant foods, and you'll notice a huge difference in how you feel and show up in the world.

Food sources with vitamin D: Our bodies depend on vitamin D to facilitate immune health, help us absorb calcium, and keep our bones healthy. Studies show that if you don't have enough vitamin D, you're at increased risk for uterine fibroids.[41]

Plant-based milks, cereal, and orange juice are usually fortified with vitamin D. And we all know we can get vitamin D from being out in the sun. Just be sure you use some sunscreen, and don't stay out

---

41. Maryam Hajhashemi, Maryam Ansari, Fedyeh Haghollahi, and Bita Eslami, "The effect of vitamin D supplementation on the size of uterine leiomyoma in women with vitamin D deficiency," *Caspian Journal of Internal Medicine* 10, no. 2 (Spring 2019): 125–131, https://www.ncbi.nlm.nih.gov/pmc/articles/PMC6619469/.

under the sun's rays for too long. Also, the light from the sun is incredibly healing for the womb in general. So, while you're out there, lift up your shirt. Let the sun's rays fall across your womb and infuse it with some energy.

Food sources with calcium: Calcium has a way of slipping out of our bodies if there isn't enough vitamin D in there to help it stay put. Vitamin D supports your body in absorbing calcium, which, in turn, will make your bones stronger. Not only that, but a study found that calcium can help ease PMS symptoms and pain during your cycle.[42]

Plant-based sources of calcium include beans, peas, lentils, broccoli, kale, brussels sprouts, cabbage, tofu, and chia seeds.

Food sources with omega-3 fatty acids: To keep the uterus healthy, be sure to add some omega-3 fatty acids to your diet. They provide the body with healthy fat and can even enhance the functioning of the reproductive system. It's a big bonus for those of us who are trying to get pregnant, or even want to just create a healthy environment in the uterus while being pregnant. Omega-3 fatty acids are also known to protect against breast cancer and other inflammatory diseases. It's even said that ingesting omega-3 fatty acids while you're breastfeeding helps enhance the health and intelligence of your baby.[43] For this one, plant-based sources of omega-3 fatty acids like walnuts, chia seeds, hempseeds, and seaweed will do the trick.

Food sources with vitamin C: If you've had a C-section, this means you have scar tissue in your abdominal area. Over time, the scar tissue can grow and form adhesions, which are thick, sticky bands that can get caught on organs. Over 90 percent of people who have had an abdominal surgery

42. Fatemeh Shobeiri, Fahimeh Ezzati Araste, Reihaneh Ebrahimi, Ensiyeh Jenabi, and Mansour Nazari, "Effect of calcium on premenstrual syndrome: A double-blind randomized clinical trial," *Obstetrics & Gynecology Science* 60, no. 1 (January 2017): 100–105, https://www.ncbi.nlm.nih.gov/pmc/articles/PMC5313351/.

43. "Here's What You Need to Know About Omega-3 While Breastfeeding," OmegaQuant, August 20, 2020, https://omegaquant.com/heres-what-you-need-to-know-about-omega-3-while-breastfeeding/.

will develop adhesions. These adhesions can cause pelvic pain, bowel obstructions, and even infertility.[44] Studies have shown that vitamin C helps reduce the formation of adhesions and enhance wound healing.[45] All my C-section mamas out there have got to give vitamin C a try. Actually, if you've had any kind of pelvic or abdominal surgery, you might also want to reach for some vitamin C. The good thing is that there are so many yummy plant-based food sources that contain vitamin C. Strawberries, oranges, mangoes, potatoes, papaya, cantaloupe, tomatoes, and pineapples—these are just some of the vegan vitamin C sources you can consume to bring healing to your body.

Nuts: Not only do nuts offer tasty snacking alternatives, but they also protect against uterine fibroids and even help prevent ovarian cancer and breast cancer.[46] Some of them—like almonds, cashews, and walnuts—also contain omega-3 fatty acids. The next time you're thinking about reaching for that bag of chips, stop for a moment and remember how much healthier your body and womb will be if you grab a handful of nuts instead.

Fruits and veggies: Although this is an obvious one, we sometimes forget the potential and power that fruits and vegetables contain within them. As they've sprung from Mother Nature herself, they're full of vibrancy and health, and putting them in our bodies will bring about endless benefits. Fruits and veggies support us in keeping all our reproductive

44. "Adhesions," Better Health Channel, last modified June 25, 2020, https://www.betterhealth.vic.gov.au/health/conditionsandtreatments/adhesions.

45. Behrouz Keleidari, Mohsen Mahmoudieh, Faranak Bahrami, Pejman Mortazavi, Reza Sari Aslani, and Seyed Alireza Toliyat, "The effect of vitamin A and vitamin C on postoperative adhesion formation: A rat model study," *Journal of Research in Medical Sciences* 19, no. 1 (January 2014): 28–32, https://www.ncbi.nlm.nih.gov/pmc/articles/PMC3963320/.

46. Karthik Kumar, "What Should I Eat If I Have Fibroid Tumors?" MedicineNet, medically reviewed May 3, 2022, https://www.medicinenet.com/what_should_i_eat_if_i_have_fibroid_tumors/article.htm; Krista Kleczewski, Claire Karlsson, and Edyth Dwyer, "Can a handful of nuts a day keep cancer away?" Cancer Prevention & Treatment Fund, http://stopcancerfund.org/p-breast-cancer/can-a-handful-of-nuts-a-day-keep-cancer-away/.

organs healthy.[47] They also bring down estrogen levels and can help keep uterine fibroids away.[48]

Fruit and vegetable consumption can also lower our risk of cancer and heart disease.[49]

You can drink your veggies if you want a major health and wellness infusion. Invest in a juicer, and it will *change your life*. You'll be able to juice raw veggies in the morning to start your day, which will give you a big boost of energy, clarity, and wellness. (My favorites to juice are cucumber, celery, and ginger.)

Whole grain foods: Aim to eat more whole grains and notice how much better your body feels. Whole grain foods are great for balancing estrogen in the body. White flours are often refined, which means they're stripped of vital nutrients and fiber. They offer empty nutritional value, which means you should limit consumption of white flour products as much as you can. Whole grain foods will skyrocket your womb health, and they're also linked to lower risk of heart disease, diabetes, and cancer.[50]

47. "Improve Your Reproductive Health with Food," Froedtert & Medical College of Wisconsin, last modified February 18, 2022, https://www.froedtert.com/stories/improve-your-reproductive-health-food.

48. Jillian Kubala, "How Your Diet Can Affect Estrogen Levels," Healthline, November 30, 2020, https://www.healthline.com/nutrition/foods-to-lower-estrogen; "Uterine Fibroids: Dos and Don'ts," WebMD, medically reviewed April 26, 2021, https://www.webmd.com/women/uterine-fibroids/uterine-fibroids-dos-and-donts.

49. Dagfinn Aune, Edward Giovannucci, Paolo Boffetta, Lars T. Fadnes, NaNa Keum, Teresa Norat, Darren C. Greenwood, Elio Riboli, Lars J. Vatten, and Serena Tonstad, "Fruit and vegetable intake and the risk of cardiovascular disease, total cancer and all-cause mortality—a systematic review and dose-response meta-analysis of prospective studies," *International Journal of Epidemiology* 46, no. 3 (June 2017): 1029–1056, https://www.ncbi.nlm.nih.gov/pmc/articles/PMC5837313/.

50. Dagfinn Aune, NaNa Keum, Edward Giovannucci, Lars T. Fadnes, Paolo Boffetta, Darren C. Greenwood, Serena Tonstad, Lars J. Vatten, Elio Riboli, and Teresa Norat, "Whole grain consumption and risk of cardiovascular disease, cancer, and all cause and cause specific mortality: systematic review and dose-response meta-analysis of prospective studies," *BMJ* 353 (June 14, 2016): i2716, https://www.bmj.com/content/353/bmj.i2716.

Water: Hydration is a healing and fundamental part of nourishing our feminine bodies. Hydration keeps us moist, flexible, and at ease. It lubricates our body and fills our womb with power and radiance. Our wombs rely on water. As we go about our lives, we are constantly losing water throughout the day. Our body system needs to be replenished with water to stay high functioning and healthy. Our wombs are also connected to the element of water. When we're pregnant, our babies are nestled and held by water within our wombs. Water symbolizes purification, transformation, and fertility. It's wildly necessary to sustain our lives on this planet. Water connects us to that flowing feminine element that vibrates in our every cell. We must tend to our bodies as if we were flowers in need of water to grow and bloom. Drink water throughout the day. Stay hydrated, and as you do, feel the power and flow of water within you.

WHAT TO KEEP OUT OF YOUR WOMB

When we consume things that aren't healthy for our wombs and bodies, we might start to feel depleted, fatigued, and out of balance. Taking in foods and drinks that create imbalance in the physical body can also affect us mentally, spiritually, and emotionally. Try to cut back on the items on this list for overall wellness.

Alcohol: We all know alcohol can cause some serious health issues for babies in utero. This shows us just how damaging alcohol is to womb health. Try to limit or completely cut out alcohol consumption, even if you're not pregnant. In a woman's body, alcohol is known to push up estrogen levels while bringing down testosterone. A recent study shows that alcohol can reduce a woman's odds of becoming pregnant.[51] Alcohol is also known to negatively impact female puberty, disrupt men-

---

51. Mohammad Yaser Anwar, Michele Marcus, and Kyra C. Taylor, "The association between alcohol intake and fecundability during menstrual cycle phases," *Human Reproduction* 36, no. 9 (September 2021): 2538–2548, https://www.ncbi.nlm.nih.gov/pmc/articles/PMC8561243/.

strual cycles, and interfere with reproductive functioning.[52] All around, it's just an absolute no.

Caffeine: Stay as far away from caffeine as you can. It can cause miscarriage in women who are pregnant.[53] It can also increase blood pressure and heart rate and cause digestive issues, anxiety, and nervousness.[54] In a world where countless people don't think they can survive without that morning cup of coffee, we've got to do better at educating ourselves on what exactly caffeine does to the body. We also need to search for more natural ways of increasing our energy, like drinking water, juicing, consuming more plant-based foods, exercising, and getting a full eight hours of sleep.

Junk food: We all know the body wants nothing to do with junk food. It's lacking in any kind of nutritional value while infusing the body with loads of calories and sugar. Keep junk food as far away from your womb as possible. Junk food increases inflammation in the body and can lead to obesity, digestive issues, cancer, and heart disease. It can also affect your mood and make you feel depressed, anxious, and foggy in the head.

Animal products: As mentioned earlier in the chapter, animal products aren't ideal when it comes to keeping our bodies healthy, well, and balanced. Meat consumption has been linked to increased odds of breast cancer and ovarian cancer.[55] Eating a lot of red meat also shows increased

52. Mary Ann Emanuele, Frederick Wezeman, and Nicholas V. Emanuele, "Alcohol's Effects on Female Reproductive Function," National Institute on Alcohol Abuse and Alcoholism, June 2003, https://pubs.niaaa.nih.gov/publications/arh26-4/274-281.htm.

53. "Couples' pre-pregnancy caffeine consumption linked to miscarriage risk," National Institutes of Health, March 24, 2016, https://www.nih.gov/news-events/news-releases/couples-pre-pregnancy-caffeine-consumption-linked-miscarriage-risk.

54. Franziska Spritzler, "9 Side Effects of Too Much Caffeine," Healthline, August 14, 2017, https://www.healthline.com/nutrition/caffeine-side-effects#TOC_TITLE_HDR_3.

55. Maryam S. Farvid, Eunyoung Cho, Wendy Y. Chen, A. Heather Eliassen, and Walter C. Willett, "Dietary protein sources in early adulthood and breast cancer incidence: prospective cohort study," BMJ 348 (June 10, 2014): g3437, https://www.bmj.com/content/348/bmj.g3437; Mary L. Carter, "Processed Meat and Hormone-related Cancers," MedPage Today, May 16, 2018, https://www.medpagetoday.com/resource-centers/focus-ovarian-cancer/processed-meat-and-hormone-related-cancers/2004.

risk for heart disease, digestive issues, high cholesterol, and even endometriosis.[56] Eating beef and other red meat can even lead to an increased risk of uterine fibroids.[57] Although our culture has been accustomed to consuming a lot of meat, you don't have to continue following the script. Try to experiment with bringing in more plant-based foods and keep a journal on how you feel as you eat this way. The results will undoubtedly speak for themselves.

Chapter 21 Takeaways

- Plant-based foods help nourish the womb and body.
- This isn't an all-or-nothing game. You don't need to be 100 percent vegan in order to get the benefits of plant-based foods. Try to incorporate vegan foods as often as you can. Maybe choose one to three days a week to be primarily plant-based.
- Keep your body and womb hydrated by drinking a lot of water.
- Stay away from alcohol, caffeine, and processed foods.

56. Ayae Yamamoto, Holly R. Harris, Allison F. Vitonis, Jorge E. Chavarro, and Stacey A. Missmer, "A prospective cohort study of meat and fish consumption and endometriosis risk," *American Journal of Obstetrics & Gynecology* 219, no. 2 (August 2019): 178.E1–178.E10, https://www.ajog.org/article/S0002-9378(18)30444-7/fulltext.

57. F. Chiaffarino, F. Parazzini, C. La Vecchia, L. Chatenoud, E. Di Cintio, S. Marsico, "Diet and uterine myomas," *Obstetrics and Gynecology* 94, no. 3 (September 1999): 395–398, https://pubmed.ncbi.nlm.nih.gov/10472866/.

Chapter 22

Womb Flow:
The Practice

"Those who flow as life flows know they need no other force."
   —*Lao Tzu*[58]

Every atom of a woman's body is encoded with the inclination to flow. At its heart, the feminine system is a fusion of ease, fluidity, and grace. There is a native rhythm that beats within the core of every woman, that stretches and bends to meet and merge with the vitality present in all women.

This isn't something we're aware of at all times. For some of us, it's not something we've ever been aware of, but something we've always yearned for—to find that natural flow state upon which our limitless potential moves and expands.

When you're in your flow, you bring all of yourself up to the surface to be expressed. You lock into your gifts and talents and find the perfect ways to put them out into the world. You bring more peace, freedom, and joy into your heart. You find your way back to the truth of what you are, to the power you've kept hidden for so long.

If our words, thoughts, actions, and feelings are out of alignment, it's a disruption of flow. But when we lock into a deep state of flow, everything is

---

58. Wayne W. Dyer, *Change Your Thoughts—Change Your Life* (New York: Hay House, 2009), 71.

in alignment. What we say, do, think, and feel all operate as one single arrow, blazing forward in one direction.

How do we get into this flow state, exactly? Not only that, but how do we maintain it so that it's not fleeting? That way, we can allow this flow state to transform our relationships, creative projects, careers, moods, and overall lives.

The answer is, through the body and the womb.

It's through movement. It's about liberating the energy in the body and womb and finding that natural vitality that will unlock our sense of flow.

Our bodies have grown too accustomed to the rhythms of the daily grind. We find ourselves, by habit, moving our bodies in the same rigid ways each day. We sit at our computers, slump our shoulders, and breathe into the chest, just like the day before. We stride down the hallway, or up the stairs, or across the cafeteria with the gait or the posture we've always used. We tackle our challenges, manage our ups and downs, and juggle our responsibilities with the same breathing patterns and physical movements we've known for years.

In working with women and experimenting with my own body, I've seen how transformational it can be to move in the ways our physical feminine selves are yearning for.

Finding your flow means breaking up patterns.

Finding your flow also means disentangling yourself from limiting habits, waking up your feminine energy, and clearing out any stuckness that might be present in the body and womb space. You can make this happen just by moving and listening to your body.

Finding flow within your body creates the conditions for your mind to take a back seat. You're no longer directing traffic and attempting to control things from your mental space. *You're going deeper.* You're listening to your internal energies, feelings, and emotions. You're allowing all of who you are to cut past the noise, drama, and empty chatter.

Finding flow is an essential part of amplifying your feminine vibration. It is the key to harmonizing the mental, physical, emotional, and spiritual parts of yourself.

This is why I created my own unique practice called Womb Flow, which supports women in finding their natural state of ease, joy, and power. Womb Flow is a deep practice that includes feminine-inspired movement, stretching, dance, and synchronized breathing.

When I toured for my first book, *Fierce Woman*, I started meeting with different women from all walks of life. I would talk a bit about my book, and began sharing deep movement practices that involved the womb and breasts. Many women would come up to me afterward, incredulous, saying they had never experienced this type of work before. They would say it had woken up something inside of them, made them feel their energy and themselves in a way they never had before.

This was when I knew.

Women are yearning to find ways back to themselves, to know the vibrant power of who and what they are. And my practices, which I've worked on creating and sharing over the past decade, could potentially help them unleash what was within. It could help them bravely plunge headfirst into what it means to claim their feminine selves and to start understanding and tending to their wombs.

And so, Womb Flow was born. It is a cumulation of my knowledge and wisdom as a women's circle facilitator, tantric educator, Kundalini Yoga teacher, and yoni steam practitioner. My heart is tied up in this work, because I've seen what it can do. I've also seen the tremendous amount of power, compassion, and resilience radiating in every woman I've ever met, despite all the challenges she has endured in life.

I want Womb Flow to be a light, a place where women can find refuge, a place where they can dare to stretch beyond any preconceived limitations. Womb Flow is a deep self-love practice, a way of honoring the wild calling that throbs inside of you. It can be practiced daily, and it should be the kind of practice that is not just done for the sake of it. It should be a practice that moves and breathes, that lives beyond the practice itself and becomes a way of living and honoring who you are.

Womb Flow Sequences

The foundation of Womb Flow features a series of exercises designed to activate and cleanse the womb. Movements that stimulate energy in the breasts and spark life throughout the body are also involved. Remember, the breasts and womb are connected and send energy back and forth between each other. The more aware you are of this connection as you flow through these practices, the deeper you'll be able to go.

Womb Flow also works a lot with the pelvis and hips, as these areas are where our feminine energy is stored. And since the spine is a major pathway through which this energy moves, Womb Flow involves a lot of movements to warm up and lubricate the spinal area.

The beauty of Womb Flow is that it's a physical, emotional, and spiritual practice. As you move and come into your feminine body, your mind will start to quiet. You'll start to clear all the cobwebs that have been keeping you from feeling bliss and joy within your body. You'll also be balancing your emotions, boosting your immunity, and getting a nice workout in the process.

I've written out a sequence of Womb Flow practices below for you to follow. However, since a written format might not always be the best substitute for physically seeing someone do the practice, I also have videos up on my website that show the exercises in detail. If you'd like to see the videos, go to rhodajordanshapiro.com/womb.

To Start

Before you begin Womb Flow, make sure you're wearing something you feel comfortable moving around in. Decide whether or not you want to play some music, or do your Womb Flow in silence. The practice works great either way. Music makes it fun and might give you a boost of energy as you do the practices; and without the music, you'll most likely go through the practices in a slower, more deeply meditative way.

The Womb Flow practices here are meant to be done in a standing position, but if you need to sit down, you can do that as well.

Before you start, take a few womb breaths as you focus on your womb.

Place your hands over your womb. Take a moment to feel your womb as the core of yourself, the place from which all movements emanate.

Now you're ready to begin.

WOMB FLOW: WARM-UP SEQUENCE

This is a set of warm-up practices to start getting present in the body and harnessing awareness for your womb.

Warm-Up 1

- Stand with your hands on your hips.
- As you inhale, open your chest and womb up toward the sky. Allow your head to naturally tilt up and face the sky as well.
- As you exhale, come back into a neutral position.
- Repeat this for one to two minutes.

Warm-Up 2

- Keep your hands on your hips.
- Lean your upper body toward the left side as you inhale. Feel the right side of the womb and body stretch and open.
- Then, exhale and come back into a neutral position.
- Repeat the same movement on the right side.
- Repeat this for one to two minutes, going back and forth from left to right.

Warm-Up 3

- Remain in a standing position if you can. But if you're unable to keep standing, please feel free to sit in a chair for this one.
- This movement involves stretching the arms up toward the sky one by one. As you do this, you will naturally feel the side of your womb opening and stretching.
- As you inhale, stretch your left hand all the way up, as if you're actually trying to reach the sky.

- As you exhale, bring the left arm down at the same time you're bringing your right arm up.
- Make sure as you stretch your arm up to the sky that you open all your fingers wide and reach up.
- And keep this going. As you inhale, the right arm goes down while the left goes up. And as you exhale, the right arm goes up and the left arm goes down. Do this for thirty seconds.
- Now switch sides. This time, start with the right hand as you inhale. And as you exhale, let the right arm come down and the left arm go up. Do this for another thirty seconds.

Womb Flow: Activations

These practices are meant to deepen your connection to your womb and that sense of flow that is innate within your body.

Womb Activation 1

- Stand up straight with your feet right next to one another. Keep your hands on your hips.
- Now, inhale and step your left foot out to the left side. At the same time you are inhaling and stepping, you also want to arch your back and feel that you are pushing your womb out. It might sound like a lot to think about at once, but synchronizing the movements and the breath will come easily to you, as you start.
- Next, as you exhale, step that left foot back to its starting position— where it was before, right next to the right foot. As you do this, be sure to bring your spine and womb back to a neutral position.
- Once you're done with that, move to the right. We're repeating the same exact movement as we did on the left side. Take an inhale as you step your right foot to the side and arch your back, pushing your womb out.
- Then take an exhale as you step your right foot back to the starting position, bringing your spine and womb back to a neutral position.

- Continue this movement, going back and forth, left to right.
- Each time you inhale and press your womb open, be sure to really *feel it*. Feel all its energy opening and expanding outward. This is your chance to wake up and supercharge your womb space. Try to be fully present and aware during this movement! Do this for at least one to two minutes.

Womb Activation 2

For this next movement, it's going to look basically the same as Womb Activation 1, except for one extra flourish...

- This time, as you inhale and step to the left, you won't just do a simple arch of your back and stick your womb out. Instead you will roll your shoulders up to your ears, press your chest forward, and tilt your chin up to the sky as you push your womb out.
- Next, without breaking up the flow of the movement, you want to exhale and step back to the center, rolling your shoulders back down, bringing your chest, spine, womb, and chin back to a neutral position. The tilting of your chest in and out should be one movement. Try not to interrupt the flow.
- Do the same thing on the right side.
- As you do this, allow your arms and hands to flow and move in whatever ways they feel inspired to.
- Continue flowing, left to right, for a couple of minutes.

The idea here isn't that you do the movement perfectly, but that you start to feel the natural sense of flow in your own body while stimulating energy in the womb. You can even close your eyes as you do this, which will help you get into your body and feel what is happening inside of you.

If all the steps and breathing just seem too confusing to you, you can even do a simple version of it. It would look like this: stay standing in one place; as you inhale, roll your shoulders up to your ears and push your womb open; as you exhale, roll your shoulders back and down, allowing your womb to go back into a neutral position.

Regardless of what version you do, go slowly here and really allow your-self to feel your body and womb. Do these activations for a few minutes.

WOMB FLOW: BREAST ACTIVATIONS

This womb-centered practice would be nothing without bringing in the energy and vibrancy of our breasts. Waking up those lively channels in the chest and heart area will wake up your body and unfurl your inner vibration.

Heart and Spine Activation

- Stand up with a straight spine. (If you're not able to stand, feel free to do this one seated in a chair.)
- Bring your palms together in front of your heart.
- Keeping your palms and hands together in front of you, inhale and shift your upper body to the left. Then exhale and shift your upper body to the right.
- Continue doing this, back and forth.
- Continue this movement for about one minute.
- Now start with the opposite side. Inhale as you move to the right, and exhale as you move to the left. Continue the movement for one minute.

The idea here is that you want to isolate the top half of your body and only let that part move. Try to keep everything from the hips on down still.

Breast Shake

- This one is done in a standing position. But if you're unable to stand, it can also be done seated.
- Take a deep inhale, and as you do, tilt your body forward and do a shoulder shake. Feel your breasts relax and release.
- Exhale and continue to shake your shoulders as you tilt your body back.
- Continue this exercise for one to two minutes.

One thing to keep in mind here is that as you're pulling back, you're not going back into a neutral position. The top of your spine is stretching out behind you while you're doing this exhale and continuing to shake out the shoulders. You should also still feel movement happening in the breasts as you do the exhale.

Figure 8 with Breasts
- As you're standing, draw a figure 8 with your breasts.
- The best way to do this is to imagine you're drawing from the center of your chest. Focus on the point in the middle of your breasts. Then, from that center point, start to draw the figure 8. Your shoulders and upper body will naturally start to create this movement.
- Allow the body to flow through this as you continue to draw the figure 8 again and again.
- Keep the lower body still.
- Do this for one to two minutes.

For this one, breathing does not need to be synchronized with the movement. Just be sure to continue your deep womb breaths into the belly.

Womb Flow: Integrations

Use these next few exercises as an opportunity to be conscious of integrating womb and heart energy together. As you do this Womb Flow practice more, you'll naturally start flowing through all the practices. But as you're just beginning, you might need some conscious reminders to integrate womb and heart. The practices here are great tools to use for mindful integration.

Figure 8 with Hips
- In a standing position, do the figure 8 from your breasts a few times.
- Now, add the lower body and make figure 8s with your hips. Let the belly button be your center point for concentration.

- From the belly button, imagine you are drawing a figure 8 in both directions, just as you're doing with the breasts. As you do this, notice your hips start to move, along with your shoulders and upper body.
- As you flow through these movements, you won't need to pay strict attention to the belly button. Let yourself feel the connection to breasts and womb as you continue to create your figure 8s. Feel the way the body naturally flows; notice how organic the motion feels throughout your body.
- Do this for a couple of minutes.

Again, there is not synchronization of breath and movement for this one. Keep doing your womb breaths, and allow the flow to overtake you.

Heel Bounce

- Stand up with your arms hanging naturally from your sides.
- Put your weight into the balls of your feet, letting your heels come slightly off the floor.
- Now, bounce up and down on your heels, allowing your body to shake. Feel your breasts and womb, and imagine they are releasing any stuck energies or emotions you might be holding on to.
- Do this for at least a minute.

Circle Dance

Feminine energy is inherently circular, operating without the need for logic or linear focus. This means the power of nature, which operates upon the foundation of cycles, can be found in our bodies. The aliveness, energy, abundance, and wildness found in women is also found in nature.

Locking into the energy of cycles within our bodies puts us in direct contact with our feminine power.

For this Circle Dance practice, which is one of my favorites, your mission is to create as many circles as you can in your body. Let the circles all spring from one another, so that your body is able to flow. Make circles with your hips, your shoulders, your head and neck. Make circles with your wrists, your arms, and your spine. Get creative, and give yourself over to the process. There is an art to this, an opportunity to let your body take full control. Notice how your body wants to make circles, and surrender to that.

As always, be sure to take your womb breaths.

You can stay in one place as you do this, or you can walk around the room. Play some music to help you stay in your flow.

Let the Circle Dance consume you for at least five minutes.

Keep Flowing

This simple Womb Flow set can be done in fifteen to twenty-five minutes. You can try the entire series or pick and choose a few exercises that really resonate with you. If you want to just do a few exercises, you can even devote a few minutes to each one and let yourself go deeper. It's your journey, so make sure it feels good to you and your body.

Again, if you want to see the practices in action and do them along with me, you can access the videos here: rhodajordanshapiro.com/womb.

You'll also find some new exercises there, if you want to learn more Womb Flow practices.

Womb Flow was designed to support the feminine body in reaching the deepest levels of expression, transmutation, and embodiment. Practice it first thing in the morning, or anytime during the day when you feel like your body needs energy, self-care, or healing. Some of the practices can really get your heart rate going, so you can even use this practice for a feminine-based way of getting a workout in! Since Womb Flow activates your body by waking up your own natural vibrancy, it's something you can always use to bring more aliveness, sensuality, confidence, joy, and peace into your day.

Once you've done the exercises, you must take the energy you've stirred up and use it out in the world. Become a living embodiment of truth, love, pleasure, joy, abundance, and sensuality. You are naturally those things already. It's just a matter of maintaining those deep joyful states and then bringing that energy into everything you do, so all your actions, your relationships, your creativity, your work—all of it becomes infused with the dynamic feminine force you are.

This energy does nobody any good just sitting dormant inside of you. Wake it up and let it move through you. Let it fill the world with something tangible and beautiful.

CHAPTER 22 TAKEAWAYS

- The ability to "be in your flow" is a gift from our feminine bodies. Once we activate a state of flow within us, everything in our lives falls into alignment.
- Practicing Womb Flow is a way of liberating the expression in your body and finding a natural state of ease and power.
- Womb Flow uses dance, synchronized breathing, feminine-inspired movement, and stretching to activate our inner potential.
- Once you've experienced the Womb Flow practices, be sure to take the energy you've awakened out into the world. Live, breathe, and move from a place of flow, and it will transform your entire life.

Conclusion

KEEP IT GOING

I've spent so many years ignoring my womb. But instead of looking back, and wondering about all the lost time and potential, I stay planted right in this moment. The present moment is the place where possibility lies, where a woman can know and feel the truth of who she is, without any constraints and hesitations.

When you stay connected to your womb, you stay connected to your inner power source. To that place inside of you where love, creativity, and energy are all intertwined.

Living your life as a Womb-Centered Woman means your every action, thought, and word is informed by love. It means you're done with playing small. You're daring to stand tall and "take up space."

Taking up space is not just limited to the physical aspect of you. You take up space when you express your voice, or when you do something kind for someone else. You take up space when you stand up for what you believe in, or when you reach out to comfort a friend who's going through a rough patch. You take up space when you go out and attack your goals like it's nobody's business. You take up space when you create something, like a baby, or a painting, or a song.

You take up space by simply being who you are, by letting the wildness inside of you unravel so that it is unleashed upon the world.

Woman, you've got power inside of you. Unlike anything the world has ever seen. You are a gift. And your presence on this planet is meaningful. You're here to love and to express your own unique magic.

If you ever forget what you are, come back to these pages to remind yourself. Do the practices and the womb breaths. Start a Womb Circle and go through this book with like-minded women who are seeking transformation and sisterhood. Take some time away from the madness of the world to sit in silence whenever you need to, so that you can find your way back to yourself again. It might take a moment, but you'll get there.

Remember that your womb and your breasts carry energies that are anything but stagnant. You can hear, feel, and experience these energies anytime you want to. You can sustain them throughout your entire day, week, month, or year. Or for the rest of your life, even.

Just stay aligned. Consciously carve out the time and space to love, honor, and be present to your body. Life goes by way too quickly for you to not pay attention to what is right there inside of you. Plug into your womb, and from there, live from the wildest depths of your heart. I dare you.

I dare you to live a life congruent to the dreams that stretch wildly across your heart.

I dare you to take up space.

I dare you to love yourself, to love your body and your womb, and to receive, with open arms, the many blessings that come pouring your way as a result.

Glossary

Castor oil: A healing vegetable oil with multiple benefits. It stimulates the circulatory system, reduces inflammation, and is incredibly healing for the womb and belly.

Cesarean: Also known as a C-section or cesarean section, this is when a surgical incision is made in the womb and abdomen so that a baby can be birthed or delivered.

Chakra: A spinning wheel of energy inside the body. There are seven main chakras that go from the base of the spine to the top of the head. Activating this positive energy is deeply healing and rejuvenating.

Dantian: "Field of elixir" in Chinese. The dantian is a central energy center in the body. The lower dantian is located in the lower abdomen and is believed to be a place of power. There are three dantians in total; the other two are in the heart and between the eyebrows.

Endometriosis: A painful condition where tissue similar to, but distinct from, the womb's inner lining is found in other areas of the body.

Fallopian tubes: Through these tubes, eggs are carried from the ovaries to the uterus every month. If an egg does get fertilized, the fallopian tubes carry the egg over to the uterus to be implanted.

Hara: This is a Japanese word that refers to the belly or lower abdomen. It is believed to be the power source of every human body.

Hysterectomy: A surgical procedure in which the womb is removed.

Menopause: A time in a woman's life when menstruation comes to an end. It happens usually between ages forty-five and fifty-five, when women have undergone twelve months with no period. It marks a transition of owning our inner wisdom and stepping into our fullest power as women.

Menstruation: The monthly blood shed from the lining of the uterus. It's an opportunity for women to align to their inner magic and creative abilities.

Ovaries: Located on either side of the womb, these two glands store and protect a woman's eggs. The ovaries make the hormones estrogen and progesterone, which play a big part in menstruation, pregnancy, and fertility.

Pranayama: An enlivening breathing practice that stems from ancient yogic practices.

Scar tissue: Thick tissue that forms in the place of healthy tissue. After injury or surgery, scar tissue forms as a way of healing the body. It's very thick, fibrous tissue that can create problems in the body, such as pain, bowel obstructions, tightness, or numbness.

Tantra: A practice of activating the senses, listening to the body, and tapping the natural vibrancy inside of ourselves, so that we can experience life in a deeper way.

Uterine fibroids: Tumors that grow in a woman's uterus. They're made up of fibrous connective tissue and smooth muscle cells, and they are usually benign.

Vagina: An inner canal that connects the uterus to the outside world. It is often only thought of during menstruation, childbirth, and sex. The vagina is the space that transmutes the womb's magic into the physical world.

Vulva: This is the outside of a woman's genitalia, and it includes the vaginal opening, labia, clitoris, and urethra.

Womb: Also known as the uterus, the womb is every woman's power source. It's an organ located in a woman's pelvis and is where our creativity, sensuality, emotions, and energy reside. The womb is the dynamic spark where creative ideas flourish. It's the place where babies are conceived, developed, and birthed from.

Womb breath: A deep conscious breath you take from deep down in your womb. Breathing this way can center you, put you in your power, and align you to your inner potential.

Wombfirmation: A way of stating affirmations and using the power of words to nourish the womb.

Womb Flow: A series of womb-nourishing practices that involve movement, breathwork, stretching, and dance. These practices are empowering and help unleash that sense of flow, self-love, and sensuality in a woman's body. Womb Flow not only impacts the womb, but it is also rejuvenating for the pelvis and reproductive organs.

Womb wrapping: The practice of wrapping one's womb with a cloth, scarf, or other wrap. It's a very soothing way to bring attention and love to the womb.

Yoni steaming: Also known as vaginal steaming or V-steaming, it involves a process of bringing the vagina over steaming water full of herbs. This brings nurturing and healing to the reproductive organs.

RESOURCES

STAY CONNECTED

For more womb practices and to stay in touch with me, go to rhoda
jordanshapiro.com/womb.

RECOMMENDED BOOKS

Fierce Woman: Wake Up Your Badass Self by Rhoda Jordan Shapiro

Sacred Woman: A Guide to Healing the Feminine Body, Mind, and Spirit by
Queen Afua

Womb Awakening: Initiatory Wisdom from the Creatrix of All Life by Azra Bertrand, MD, and Seren Bertrand

*Code Red: Know Your Flow, Unlock Your Superpowers, and Create a Bloody
Amazing Life. Period.* by Lisa Lister

*Women's Bodies, Women's Wisdom: Creating Physical and Emotional Health and
Healing* by Christiane Northrup, MD

Tao Tantric Arts for Women: Cultivating Sexual Energy, Love, and Spirit by
Minke de Vos

Breath by James Nestor

SCAR TISSUE RESOURCES

Microcurrent Therapy—The Dolphin Neurostim Professional Scar Release Kit contains two microcurrent devices that are highly effective for softening scar tissue: https://www.dolphinmps.com/product/dolphin-neurostim-professional-ddk/.

Scar Tissue Release Therapy—If you're ever anywhere near Sebastopol, California, get yourself over to Ananda Fierro's Scar Tissue Release Therapy. She provides hands-on myofascial release work, while also using microcurrent therapy to help release scar tissue. I've worked with her, and she's just amazing at what she does. Not only that, but she truly cares. https://www.scartissuereleasetherapy.com.

Abdominal Adhesion Program—This is an online course for self-massage on abdominal adhesions. It's an empowering way of taking matters into your own hands (literally) and massaging your scar tissue. The woman who teaches it, Isabel Spradlin, is an amazing guide and breaks things down in a very easy-to-follow format. I've taken the course and often use her techniques. https://abdominaladhesiontreatment.com/recover/.

BIBLIOGRAPHY

Abrams, Abiola. *African Goddess Initiation: Sacred Rituals for Self-Love, Prosperity, and Joy.* New York: Hay House, 2021.

Ackerman, Diane. *A Natural History of the Senses.* New York: Vintage, 1991.

"Adhesions." Better Health Channel. Last modified June 25, 2020. https://www.betterhealth.vic.gov.au/health/conditionsandtreatments/adhesions.

Afua, Queen. *Sacred Woman: A Guide to Healing the Feminine Body, Mind, and Spirit.* New York: One World, 2000.

Ajala, Iya Olosunde. *Yoni Steam: Divine Feminine Hygiene.* Self-published, 2015.

Angelou, Maya. *I Know Why the Caged Bird Sings.* New York: Random House, 1969.

Anwar, Mohammad Yaser, Michele Marcus, and Kyra C. Taylor. "The association between alcohol intake and fecundability during menstrual cycle phases." *Human Reproduction* 36, no. 9 (September 2021): 2538–2548. https://www.ncbi.nlm.nih.gov/pmc/articles/PMC8561243/.

Araki, Miyuki, Shota Nishitani, Keisho Ushimaru, Hideaki Masuzaki, Kazuyo Oishi, and Kazuyuki Shinohara. "Fetal response to induced maternal emotions." *The Journal of Physiological Sciences* 60 (February 2010): 213–220. https://jps.biomedcentral.com/articles/10.1007 /s12576-010-0087-x.

Aune, Dagfinn, Edward Giovannucci, Paolo Boffetta, Lars T. Fadnes, NaNa Keum, Teresa Norat, Darren C. Greenwood, Elio Riboli, Lars J. Vatten, and Serena Tonstad. "Fruit and vegetable intake and the risk of cardiovascular disease, total cancer and all-cause mortality—a systematic review and dose-response meta-analysis of prospective studies." *International Journal of Epidemiology* 46, no. 3 (June 2017): 1029–1056. https://www .ncbi.nlm.nih.gov/pmc/articles/PMC5837313/.

Aune, Dagfinn, NaNa Keum, Edward Giovannucci, Lars T. Fadnes, Paolo Boffetta, Darren C. Greenwood, Serena Tonstad, Lars J. Vatten, Elio Riboli, and Teresa Norat. "Whole grain consumption and risk of cardiovascular disease, cancer, and all cause and cause specific mortality: systematic review and dose-response meta-analysis of prospective studies." *BMJ* 353 (June 14, 2016): i2716. https://www.bmj.com/content/353/bmj .i2716.

Bertrand, Azra, and Seren Bertrand. *Womb Awakening: Initiary Wisdom from the Creatrix of All Life*. Vermont: Bear & Company, 2017.

Carter, Mary L. "Processed Meat and Hormone-related Cancers." MedPage Today. May 16, 2018. https://www.medpagetoday.com/resource-centers /focus-ovarian-cancer/processed-meat-and-hormone-related-cancers /2004.

Chen, Lijun, Jingjing Qu, Tianli Cheng, Xin Chen, and Charlie Xiang. "Menstrual blood-derived stem cells: toward therapeutic mechanisms, novel strategies, and future perspectives in the treatment of diseases." *Stem Cell Research & Therapy* 10 (December 2019): 406. https://stemcellres.biomed central.com/articles/10.1186/s13287-019-1503-7.

"Chhaupadi and menstruation taboos." Action Aid. Last modified May 23, 2022. https://www.actionaid.org.uk/our-work/period-poverty /chhaupadi-and-menstruation-taboos.

Chiaffarino, F., F. Parazzini, C. La Vecchia, L. Chatenoud, E. Di Cintio, S. Marsico. "Diet and uterine myomas." *Obstetrics and Gynecology* 94, no. 3 (September 1999): 395–398. https://pubmed.ncbi.nlm.nih.gov /10472866/.

Chopra, Deepak. Facebook. December 9, 2011. https://www.facebook.com /DeepakChopra/posts/language-creates-reality-words-have-power-speak -always-to-create-joy/10150435500685665/.

Cohut, Maria. "Menstrual Cycles and Lunar Cycles: Is There a Link?" Medical News Today. February 12, 2021. https://www.medicalnewstoday.com /articles/menstrual-cycles-and-lunar-cycles-is-there-a-link.

"Couples' pre-pregnancy caffeine consumption linked to miscarriage risk." National Institutes of Health. March 24, 2016. https://www.nih.gov /news-events/news-releases/couples-pre-pregnancy-caffeine -consumption-linked-miscarriage-risk.

"Devastatingly pervasive: 1 in 3 women globally experience violence." World Health Organization. March 9, 2021. https://www.who.int/news/item /09-03-2021-devastatingly-pervasive-1-in-3-women-globally-experience -violence.

Dyer, Wayne W. *Change Your Thoughts—Change Your Life: Living the Wisdom of the Tao.* New York: Hay House, 2009.

Dylan, Mystic. *The Witch's Guide to Manifestation: Witchcraft for the Life You Want.* Emeryville: Rockridge Press, 2021.

Emanuele, Mary Ann, Frederick Wezeman, and Nicholas V. Emanuele. "Alcohol's Effects on Female Reproductive Function." National Institute on Alcohol Abuse and Alcoholism. June 2003. https://pubs.niaaa.nih.gov /publications/arh26-4/274-281.htm.

England, Pam, and Rob Horowitz. *Birthing from Within: An Extra-Ordinary Guide to Childbirth Preparation.* New Mexico: Partera Press, 1998.

Farvid, Maryam S., Eunyoung Cho, Wendy Y. Chen, A. Heather Eliassen, and Walter C. Willett. "Dietary protein sources in early adulthood and breast cancer incidence: prospective cohort study." *BMJ* 348 (June 10, 2014): g3437. https://www.bmj.com/content/348/bmj.g3437.

Genkinger, Jeanine M., and Anita Koushik. "Meat Consumption and Cancer Risk." *PLoS Medicine* 4, no. 12 (December 2007): e345. https://www.ncbi.nlm.nih.gov/pmc/articles/PMC2121650/.

Green, Susan. "Violence Against Black Women—Many Types, Far-reaching Effects." Institute for Women's Policy Research. July 13, 2017. https://iwpr.org/iwpr-issues/race-ethnicity-gender-and-economy/violence-against-black-women-many-types-far-reaching-effects/.

Hahn, Thich Nhat. "The Way Out Is In." April 15, 2014. *Thich Nhat Hanh Dharma Talks*. Podcast. Audio, 1:47.

Hajhashemi, Maryam, Maryam Ansari, Fedyeh Haghollahi, and Bita Eslami. "The effect of vitamin D supplementation on the size of uterine leiomyoma in women with vitamin D deficiency." *Caspian Journal of Internal Medicine* 10, no. 2 (Spring 2019): 125–131. https://www.ncbi.nlm.nih.gov/pmc/articles/PMC6619469/.

"Here's What You Need to Know About Omega-3 While Breastfeeding." OmegaQuant. August 20, 2020. https://omegaquant.com/heres-what-you-need-to-know-about-omega-3-while-breastfeeding/.

Hurston, Zora Neale. *Dust Tracks on a Road: An Autobiography*. New York: HarperCollins, 1996.

"Improve Your Reproductive Health with Food." Froedtert & Medical College of Wisconsin. Last modified February 18, 2022. https://www.froedtert.com/stories/improve-your-reproductive-health-food.

Kearney, Melissa S., and Phillip Levine. "Will births in the US rebound? Probably not." The Brookings Institution. May 24, 2021. https://www.brookings.edu/blog/up-front/2021/05/24/will-births-in-the-us-rebound-probably-not/.

Keleidari, Behrouz, Mohsen Mahmoudieh, Faranak Bahrami, Pejman Mortazavi, Reza Sari Aslani, and Seyed Alireza Toliyat. "The effect of vitamin A and vitamin C on postoperative adhesion formation: A rat model study." *Journal of Research in Medical Sciences* 19, no. 1 (January 2014): 28–32. https://www.ncbi.nlm.nih.gov/pmc/articles/PMC3963320/.

Keltner, Dacher. "Hands On Research: The Science of Touch." *Greater Good Magazine*. September 29, 2010. https://greatergood.berkeley.edu/article /item/hands_on_research.

"Key Statistics for Breast Cancer." American Cancer Society. Last modified January 12, 2022. https://www.cancer.org/cancer/breast-cancer/about /how-common-is-breast-cancer.html.

Kleczewski, Krista, Claire Karlsson, and Edyth Dwyer. "Can a handful of nuts a day keep cancer away?" Cancer Prevention & Treatment Fund. http://stopcancerfund.org/p-breast-cancer/can-a-handful-of-nuts-a-day -keep-cancer-away/.

Koebele, Stephanie V., et al. "Hysterectomy Uniquely Impacts Spatial Memory in a Rat Model: A Role for the Nonpregnant Uterus in Cognitive Processes." *Endocrinology* 160, no. 1 (January 2019): 1–19.

Kubala, Jillian. "How Your Diet Can Affect Estrogen Levels." Healthline. November 30, 2020. https://www.healthline.com/nutrition/foods-to -lower-estrogen.

Kumar, Karthik. "What Should I Eat If I Have Fibroid Tumors?" MedicineNet. Medically reviewed May 3, 2022. https://www.medicinenet.com /what_should_i_eat_if_i_have_fibroid_tumors/article.htm.

"Latest global cancer data: Cancer burden rises to 19.3 million new cases and 10.0 million cancer deaths in 2020." International Agency for Research on Cancer. December 15, 2020. https://www.iarc.who.int/wp-content /uploads/2020/12/pr292_E.pdf.

Lister, Lisa. *Love Your Lady Landscape: Trust Your Gut, Care for 'Down There' and Reclaim Your Fierce and Feminine SHE Power*. London: Hay House, 2016.

Lynn, Tanya. *The Art of Leading Circle: How to Fill, Lead, and Grow a Women's Circle*. New Fern Publishing, 2020.

Mak, Pawel, Kinga Wojcik, Lukasz Wicherek, Piotr Suder, and Adam Dubin. "Antibacterial hemoglobin peptides in human menstrual blood." *Peptides* 25, no. 11 (November 2004): 1839–1847. https://pubmed.ncbi.nlm.nih .gov/15501514/.

Morales, Jessica I. "The Heart's Electromagnetic Field Is Your Superpower." *Psychology Today*. November 29, 2020. https://www.psychologytoday .com/us/blog/building-the-habit-hero/202011/the-hearts -electromagnetic-field-is-your-superpower.

National Oceanic and Atmospheric Administration. "How much of the ocean have we explored?" US Department of Commerce. Last modified February 26, 2021. https://oceanservice.noaa.gov/facts/exploration .html.

Nestor, James. *Breath*. New York: Riverhead Books, 2020.

Northrup, Christiane. *Women's Bodies, Women's Wisdom: Creating Physical and Emotional Health and Healing*. 5th ed. New York: Bantam Books, 2020.

Perry, Susan. "1 in 5 hysterectomies in U.S. may be unnecessary, study finds." *MinnPost*. January 18, 2015. https://www.minnpost.com/second-opinion /2015/01/1-5-hysterectomies-us-may-be-unnecessary-study-finds/.

"Red and processed meat linked to increased risk of heart disease, Oxford study shows." University of Oxford. July 21, 2021. https://www.ox.ac.uk /news/2021-07-21-red-and-processed-meat-linked-increased-risk-heart -disease-oxford-study-shows.

Richardson, Diana. *Tantric Orgasm for Women*. Vermont: Destiny Books, 2004.

Sandman, Curt A., Elysia Poggi Davis, and Laura M. Glynn. "Prescient Human Fetuses Thrive." *Psychological Science* 23, no.1 (January 2012): 93–100.

Seppälä, Emma. "Breathing: The Little Known Secret to Peace of Mind." *Psychology Today*. April 15, 2013. https://www.psychologytoday.com/us /blog/feeling-it/201304/breathing-the-little-known-secret-peace-mind.

Shobeiri, Fatemeh, Fahimeh Ezzati Araste, Reihaneh Ebrahimi, Ensiyeh Jenabi, and Mansour Nazari. "Effect of calcium on premenstrual syndrome: A double-blind randomized clinical trial." *Obstetrics & Gynecology Science* 60, no. 1 (January 2017): 100–105. https://www.ncbi.nlm.nih.gov/pmc /articles/PMC5313351/.

Spritzler, Franziska. "9 Side Effects of Too Much Caffeine." Healthline. August 14, 2017. https://www.healthline.com/nutrition/caffeine-side-effects#TOC_TITLE_HDR_3.

Teish, Luisah. *Jambalaya: The Natural Woman's Book of Personal Charms and Practical Rituals*. New York: HarperCollins, 1985.

US Weekly Staff. "Gwyneth Paltrow Gets Vaginal Steam at Spa, Preaches its Virtues on Goop." *US Weekly*. January 29, 2015. https://www.usmagazine.com/stylish/news/gwyneth-paltrow-gets-vagina-steam-at-spa-preaches-its-virtues-on-goop-2015291/.

"Uterine Fibroids: Dos and Don'ts." WebMD. Medically reviewed April 26, 2021. https://www.webmd.com/women/uterine-fibroids/uterine-fibroids-dos-and-donts.

Vos, Minke de. *Tao Tantric Arts for Women: Cultivating Sexual Energy, Love, and Spirit*. Vermont: Destiny Books, 2016.

World Health Organization. "Caesarean section rates continue to rise, amid growing inequalities in access." World Health Organization. June 16, 2021. https://www.who.int/news/item/16-06-2021-caesarean-section-rates-continue-to-rise-amid-growing-inequalities-in-access.

Yamamoto, Ayae, Holly R. Harris, Allison F. Vitonis, Jorge E. Chavarro, and Stacey A. Missmer. "A prospective cohort study of meat and fish consumption and endometriosis risk." *American Journal of Obstetrics & Gynecology* 219, no. 2 (August 2019): 178.E1–178.E10. https://www.ajog.org/article/S0002-9378(18)30444-7/fulltext.

ACKNOWLEDGMENTS

This book has been alive in my heart for so long. It feels good to finally have the words written and out in the world. I wouldn't have been able to do it without the support of so many amazing individuals.

Thank you to the team at Llewellyn for all your vision and support. I'm so grateful to Angela Wix and Sami Sherratt; thank you both for working your magic and putting love and care into my book.

I also want to thank my family. My heart is spilling over with gratitude for my kids, Benny and Henry; you both bring so much joy and inspiration into my life! Thank you for your love and support as I wrote this book. I know you're both still waiting for me to write a children's book; don't worry, I'm going to get to it!

I am immensely grateful for my husband, Eric. I can't think of anyone who has supported me and believed in me more than you. Thank you for being on this adventure with me, and for always being someone I can deeply trust and depend on for absolutely anything. I know there is still so much to look forward to on this journey together. I love you!

Thank you to the many spiritual teachers I've been blessed to know on my path. Your wisdom has fortified my life and deepened my commitment to the work I do. Thank you to Iya Olosunde Ajala for all your passion and dedication to healing women's wombs. I'm grateful to have been your student, and to have learned so much from you about womb care and yoni steaming. And big thanks to Melissa Habibi for your fierce love for liberating the feminine, and for helping me align to myself as a priestess. Your work is rich in my heart. Thank you also to Guru Vishnu, Shawn Roop, and Charu Morgan for your precious teachings. I'm so honored to have worked with all of you.

Thank you to Ananda Fierro for helping me heal my womb and belly. The scar tissue release therapy you do is *so* important. Thank you for stepping up and doing this meaningful work!

I appreciate Heather Mayer for being my doula and helping me navigate all the tough moments of labor and childbirth. I couldn't have birthed my second son naturally without you. I will forever be grateful for your strength, your nurturing words, and your support.

And, of course, I cannot forget to thank all the nurses and doctors who have taken care of me during several different hospital visits, as I was struggling from the effects of scar tissue. My life was literally in your hands. And I'm so grateful for all the time, care, and energy all of you put into me. You are a big part of my womb journey.

I'm grateful to my family for connecting me to the past. Keeping our connection to our ancestors and heritage is deeply important, and I'm so appreciative to my family for taking the time to share history with me. It has been both healing and refreshing for my womb and heart. A big thank-you to Nannie (my Aunt Anna). Nannie, I'm grateful for all our conversations and for the ways in which you've shown up for me. You're always there to cheer me on, and it means so much to me.

I give thanks to my Auntie Vilma, whose strength and energy I truly admire. You are one of a kind, Auntie, and I appreciate you!

Major gratitude and love also go out to my siblings, Phyllis Kletke and Stanley Jordan, who have both filled my life with so much laughter and love. There's no one like you both in the world, and I'm grateful to share a bond with you!

Thank you to my cousin Diana Jordan for always reaching out with support and love! Cousin, your own womb journey has inspired me so much; you are a true warrioress.

A big thank-you to all my amazing friends who never hesitate to be there for me. I can't mention them all here, but I did want to thank my friend Jessika Manuel for her endless support over the years. I cherish our friendship so much, and have always felt so connected to you. You're an exceptional photographer, and I'm so thrilled you did the author photo for my books!

Thank you to my dear friend Naomi La Cosse Morineau, who is always there to shower me with good vibes and positivity. I'm also grateful for my friend Jenn Torai for being such a fountain of support in everything I do. Thank you to Eva Pontillas—you empower me to always be who I am and shine my light. Thank you to Ute Ben Himane for assisting me with my work and keeping things running smoothly for these last several years. I'm so grateful for you and the friendship we have.

Again, I just can't name every friend who has impacted me, because there are so many. A big thank-you to all my goddess sisters who have been there for me over the years. Sisterhood has shaped me tremendously, and this book would not have been possible if not for all of you.

Thank you to my East Coast parents, my in-laws Nita and Jeff Shapiro. You've welcomed me into your family with open arms and shown me so much love and support over the years. A big thank-you, also, to Stephanie Tuzzeo; I'm so grateful to have such a thoughtful and amazing sister-in-law! Thank you for showing me sisterhood over the years.

Thank you to my dad, who has blessed my life with so much wisdom, warmth, and love. I don't know how I ended up so fortunate to have a dad like you. You meant the world to me, and you still do. I miss you *every single day*.

Thank you to my mom, a.k.a. Ma Mere, whose love is always a constant. Ma Mere, I'm so grateful to you for carrying me in your womb and giving birth to me! Thank you for blessing my life with your giving and caring nature. I love you, and I'm grateful to be your daughter.

Finally, thank you to all my ancestors. I dream about you all the time. I try to imagine you, to understand all the challenges you faced. I know that my life would not be possible if not for each and every single one of you. This life is a gift, and I will live it every day in honor of you.

TO WRITE TO THE AUTHOR

If you wish to contact the author or would like more information about this book, please write to the author in care of Llewellyn Worldwide Ltd. and we will forward your request. Both the author and the publisher appreciate hearing from you and learning of your enjoyment of this book and how it has helped you. Llewellyn Worldwide Ltd. cannot guarantee that every letter written to the author can be answered, but all will be forwarded. Please write to:

Rhoda Jordan Shapiro
℅ Llewellyn Worldwide
2143 Wooddale Drive
Woodbury, MN 55125-2989

Please enclose a self-addressed stamped envelope for reply,
or $1.00 to cover costs. If outside the U.S.A., enclose
an international postal reply coupon.

Many of Llewellyn's authors have websites with additional
information and resources. For more information,
please visit our website at http://www.llewellyn.com.